THE
HISTORY
OF
AMERICAN
NURSING

Edited by
Susan Reverby, Wellesley College

A GARLAND SERIES

ETHICS FOR MODERN NURSES

Katharine J. Densford
Millard S. Everett

GARLAND PUBLISHING, INC.
NEW YORK • LONDON
1984

For a complete list of the titles in this series see the final pages of this volume.

This facsimile was made from a copy in the Yale University School of Nursing Library.

Library of Congress Cataloging in Publication Data

Densford, Katharine J. (Katharine Jane), 1890-
  Ethics for modern nurses.

  (The History of American nursing)
  Reprint. Originally published: Philadelphia ; Saunders, 1946.
  Includes bibliographies and index.
  1. Nursing ethics. 2. Medical ethics. I. Everett, Millard
S. (Millard Spencer), 1897-   . II. Title. III. Series.
[DNLM: 1. Ethics, Nursing. WY 85 D413e]
RT85.D4   1984   610.73′06′9   83-49137
ISBN 0-8240-6510-7 (alk. paper)

The volumes in this series are printed on acid-free, 250-year-life paper.

Printed in the United States of America

Ethics

FOR MODERN NURSES

Professional Adjustments I

KATHARINE J. DENSFORD, M.A., R.N., D.Sc.

Director, The School of Nursing, University of Minnesota

MILLARD S. EVERETT, Ph.D.

Assistant Professor of Philosophy, University of Minnesota

W. B. SAUNDERS COMPANY

PHILADELPHIA AND LONDON

1946

Foreword

As one of the vital health professions, nursing today has a special significance as well as new responsibilities and outstanding opportunities. Spectacular advances in all fields of science are being translated into everyday living. Since the practice of nursing is the operation of principles of the social, biologic, and physical sciences, our profession will play an important part in helping to apply new knowledge, to create a new pattern of life, and to guarantee that the means of attaining optimum health are available to everyone.

Nursing has always been, and will always be, a service profession whose motives spring from humanitarian impulses. A dynamic profession, it offers deep satisfaction to young people who are impelled to understand the workings of science and to make principles function in human activity.

Nursing is creative. The mediums with which the nurse deals are human welfare and comfort. Nursing is dramatic. The nurse is the custodian of life from birth to death. She understands the realities of life and is above cynicism. Seldom does she find a situation in which she can do no good. Under her knowing and skilled ministrations, hardships lose their hopelessness.

Since it is woman's part to create and heal and comfort, nursing is one of the most rewarding vocations open to women. The nurse's experiences deepen the meaning of her life and enrich its texture, challenging her best potentialities. Learning to minister to human beings in need, to aid the sick, the suffering, and the injured, makes a difference in all her adjustments to basic human problems. Being at once womanly and scientific, nursing today is a profession for women of character and capacity, women who will promote progress in a new civilization based on democratic principles. Preparation for nursing is more than preparation for a professional career; it is preparation for living as an intelligent citizen, as wife and homemaker.

The demand for superior care of the patient has emerged in bold relief against a national backdrop of awareness of community nursing needs. In assembling the material for this book, the authors have kept constantly before them these vital questions: How can we guide young people to the full realization of their potentialities in this most rewarding of professions? What mental and spiritual equipment do they need to assure them their rightful place in a profession united in purpose and ideals? What must they learn, what can they do, to help mankind achieve optimum health and happiness?

The answers to these questions will provide serviceable tools for all students of nursing. Use them wisely, with skilled hands, cool heads, and warm hearts, so that yours will be a distinguished contribution to a proud and honorable profession.

LUCILE PETRY, R.N.

Director, Division of Nurse Education,
United States Public Health Service.

Preface

W HEN A STUDENT enters a school of nursing, she has many problems. Among them are two of prime importance. One concerns her initial adjustment to the new environment. The other is inherent in the first. It has to do with the development of a philosophy of life—the formulation and application of principles of conduct. *Ethics for Modern Nurses* is designed to deal with both of these problems.

Part I concerns itself primarily with helping the young student to adjust as quickly and as satisfactorily as possible to her new environment. It provides orientation in school, hospital, and the profession of nursing in general. Although the suggestions offered are applicable throughout the nurse's career, they are intended to be of special help to the entering student in making her initial adjustments.

Part II deals with the broader aspects of ethics. It discusses the moral principles involved in purposeful, satisfying, useful living. By examining several fundamentally different philosophies of conduct, the student comes to understand more clearly her own moral choices as well as those of others. This fosters tolerance. At the same time, sympathetic understanding and tolerance are not confused with indifference, but positive aid is given to those who wish to apply modern, common-sense ethical methods to the solution of personal, professional, and social problems. In the general confusion of global thinking and of post-war reconstruction, the not-knowing-what-to-think and the being-puzzled-to-tell-what's-right cannot but disturb everyone. If this portion of the book helps the young student in some measure to think through these perplexities to constructive conclusions, it will have fulfilled its purpose.

The text is designed for the use of either nurse students in schools of nursing or pre-nursing students in colleges and universities. It is not limited to ethics of nursing in any narrow sense. Indeed, Part II is broad enough to serve also as an introduction to social studies for those schools that have little or no time for the teaching of social sciences.

The authors, who themselves may occasionally hold different opinions on philosophical and religious questions, have written the book with a view to meeting the need of those schools, both large and small, which aim at the teaching of principles rather than of specific rules of conduct. While a few rules are suggested, this type of treatment is not stressed. It is felt that the student learns much of the details of desirable conduct in the varied situations of actual nursing practice, both in introductory courses and in the various clinical nursing services. Provision is made at the end of each chapter for the discussion of specific situations, though it is preferable that the discussion in each class center around actual problems which are confronting the students from day to day.

Teachers in nursing schools affiliated with religious organizations will find the point of view of the text to be consistent with the best elements in our religious tradition. The fact that there is no conflict between liberal ethics and a truly religious spirit is made clear.

In writing a book of this sort one is indebted to numberless persons—to students, friends, and colleagues. Advice and help have come from many. We wish especially to express our gratitude to Professor Wayne A. R. Leys, Roosevelt College, Chicago, for invaluable assistance in revising the second part of the manuscript; to Professor George P. Conger, University of Minnesota, for reading the manuscript and making a number of helpful criticisms; to Laura R. Logan, Director, St. Louis City Hospital School of Nursing and Nursing Service; to Mary A. Hinckley, Instructor, Hyde Park High School, Chicago; to Lucile Petry, Director of Nurse Education Division, U. S. Public Health Service; and to the following members of the University of Minnesota School of Nursing faculty—Ruth Harrington and Myrtle Hodgkins Coe—for reading portions of the text and for offering suggestions both as to the text itself and as to the bibliography and questions.

K. J. DENSFORD
M. S. EVERETT

January, 1946

Contents

PART II. PERSONAL, PROFESSIONAL AND SOCIAL ETHICS

PART I. STUDENT ADJUSTMENTS

I

Your Future and the Future of Nursing

You have chosen nursing as your profession. And you are to be congratulated upon your choice. When we say this, we do so, not in the indiscriminate way in which commencement orators bestow their blessing on all alike who are entering upon careers, but rather we congratulate you with a genuine belief in the future of nursing. Our belief in the future of nursing represents a reasoned faith in the future of mankind in general. The history of civilization is inseparable from the history of nursing, and the advancement of the one contributes to the advancement of the other.

If we believe that a rational political and economic order will eventually come out of the chaos of the recent past, then we can be sure that nursing will occupy a prominent place in such an order. As the world grows more humane and learns how to put its humanity into practice, there will not only be a good and honored position waiting for everyone who has the desire and the ability to become a nurse, but the nursing profession will be in keen competition with other professions to recruit as many of the intelligent, capable, and trustworthy women, and men too, as it will urgently need.

In a society in which people would have purchasing power sufficient to obtain all the medical and nursing services they needed, as well as an abundance of other goods, the most pressing problem would be the shortage of talent. There would not be enough highly skilled workers to go around. Graduates in almost any field of study, instead of being worried for fear of not getting a job, would have the new experience of being sought after and being able to choose the best of several propositions. That is as it should be, and will be sometime, we hope.

But as things are, we have known something approaching

1

this ideal employment situation only under the boom conditions of war. In the first World War the demand for nurses was greatly increased. In the second World War approximately 65,000 applicants were admitted to schools of nursing in the academic year 1944–1945 as against 38,113 in the calendar year 1940, and about $60,000,000 were appropriated by Congress for nursing education as compared with $1,800,000 in 1941. That sort of thing is to be expected during war, for members of the armed forces require medical attention which they would not have occasion for in ordinary times, and many receive nursing services which they could not afford in private life. But what are the prospects for the nursing profession in time of peace? What does the record show?

It shows that even in the prosperous twenties employment conditions were far from ideal. In some places (the state of New York, for example) almost twice as many nurses were being graduated as could be absorbed. Hospitals were no longer able to employ all the graduates of their own schools available for "special duty" nursing, not to mention the nurses whom they had previously drawn from outside registries. In 1928 nurses' registries were almost unanimous in stating that there were too many nurses and that they did not want any more nurses to move to their cities.

But if unemployment existed at the peak of prosperity, it is obvious that the problem would become much worse in the ensuing depression. In 1934 professional registries reported that 12 per cent of the nurses on call were totally unemployed each month and only 25 per cent of the nurses reported twenty or more days of employment each month. With improvement in economic conditions in 1936, two per cent of nurses on call were totally unemployed each month but there were still only 34 per cent employed twenty days or more—a situation which fails markedly in giving nurses in private practice a sense of financial security.

Hence, one who is pessimistically inclined might conclude that all the record shows is that nursing has its ups and downs and that during peace time it is far from being up. Accordingly, it would seem unfair to the student to present too rosy a picture of her future in the nursing profession. Honest realism should make us grant that the pessimist *may* be right. We may muddle along for years after the war, hoping that somehow matters will adjust themselves automatically and save us the trouble of taking the steps that will be required to maintain full employment. If the future is like the past, there will be many unemployed, many on relief, and many doing makeshift work. And nurses will be among these unemployed. Yet, if these dire predictions prove true, there is this consolation, such as it is: that the nursing profession will be no worse off than many another one. In other words, as long as basic economic problems remain unsolved, no one can promise anything with certainty for any occupation.

Having paid our respects to such pessimism, let us see what may be said on the brighter side. In the first place, the future is not necessarily like the past. History is a development rather than just a repetition of ups and downs that get us nowhere. There is some reason to believe that there are forces operating which may come to a head sooner than we expect and unite us in a determination to solve the unemployment problem. It takes time for a nation which has enjoyed easy, unplanned prosperity in the past to convince itself that capitalism will never again work automatically and bring us prosperity, as it once did, without the aid of the government. The depression of the thirties went a long way toward teaching us that lesson, but the lesson was too new for most people to grasp even after much suffering. We did learn, however, that when an economic decline is obviously setting in, we must do something about it through our government. Hence, in this post-war period we are more prepared to act promptly.

How may this affect nursing? In this way. If the government must spend huge sums of money in order to distribute purchasing power and thus help capitalism to function, then it is certain that the public will demand that the money be spent on badly needed social services rather than on "boondoggling." And medical care will be one of the first of such services to occur to us. With more and more public consciousness of the need of medical attention for underprivileged sections of the population, people will naturally say that if the government has to spend billions, let some of this go into health services. That will mean more work for doctors and nurses.

Or, if in some other way our government succeeds in solving the unemployment problem and establishing a fairly high level of living, a greater demand for nurses will result. This may be seen from the following figures which show the relation between economic status and the use of private duty nurses in 1929:

> Among families with incomes of less than $1,200 a year, less than 6 per cent of hospital patients employed private duty nurses.
> Among families with incomes from $1,200–$2,000 a year, the ratio increased to 12 per cent.
> Among families with incomes from $2,000–$5,000 a year, the ratio was 40 per cent.
> Among families with incomes of more than $10,000, the ratio was 69 per cent.*

If the two-thirds of all families which were receiving less than $2,000 a year in 1929 could have been raised to a level of $2,000 incomes, the number of nurses in private practice required by the nation would have been about doubled. And this would represent only the increase in the demand for nurses if all families were given an income which, according to the U.S. Department of Labor, would provide merely the minimum essentials of health and decency at the price level of 1929. If we ever achieve something better than a minimum for everyone, then the number of nurses required would be still further increased.

There are other ways also of showing that the nursing profession is on an ascending curve of growth. As civilization develops, the benefits of science, particularly medical science, are extended to larger and larger sections of the population. At present there are still many gaps to be filled before we can say that the democratic doctrine of equality has been applied to all sections of our country as regards medicine and nursing. For example, there are about three times as many nurses per

* *Facts about Nursing.* Published by the Nursing Information Bureau of the American Nurses Association, New York, 1941.

100,000 persons in the New England and in the Pacific States as in the East South Central and West South Central States. Similarly cities have a much larger number of nurses to draw upon than do rural areas. In 1930 "in the borough of Manhattan in New York City one out of every 234 people was an active graduate nurse" while "in Schoharie County," New York, "there were only four registered nurses" in the entire county, "or one for every 5,391 people." In Shreveport, Louisiana, there was a "registered nurse for every 171 white people" while "in 26 (rural) parishes with a total of nearly 244,000 white persons, there was no record of a single active graduate nurse."* The Negroes fared even worse than the poor whites in the rural areas. In 1937 there was one public health nurse for every 7,000 of the entire population of the United States, but for Negroes there was only one for every 20,000. Obviously, when all the underprivileged segments of the American people are allowed to have their just share in the benefits of civilization, this will mean a great increase in demand for nurses.

Again, when we consider the amazing increase in enrollments in hospitalization insurance plans since the movement was initiated by the Baylor University Hospital at Dallas, Texas, in 1929, it is clear that many persons are now making use of hospitals and nursing services who formerly went without these except in the most extreme emergencies. In a little over one decade the number enrolled in group hospitalization grew to more than ten million and is still increasing. In the early part of the twentieth century when surgery was still in a stage at which there were many failures and hospital service was far from adequate, most people had a dread of hospitals. They often felt, as they saw one of their family carried out to a hospital ambulance, that this was almost the same as being carried out to a hearse. But this is changing and hospitals now inspire warmer and friendlier associations in the mind of the public. The hospital is the place where people choose to be, if they have the means, even in the case of minor illnesses.

There is also a growth in steady, all-year-around employment

* Brown, Esther Lucille. Nursing as a Profession, 2d Ed., page 101 (Published by Russell Sage Foundation).

for nurses as indicated by the increase in normal times in the number of institutional nurses. In 1927 three-fourths of all hospitals did not employ a single graduate nurse for general care. By 1937 only 10 per cent of the hospitals maintained such a low standard of service for the public. In 1941 the number of nurses engaged in institutional and public health nursing amounted to considerably more than half of all registered nurses. In the period between 1931 and 1941 (when the Social Security Act was put into effect), the number of public health nurses increased 30 per cent to a total of 24,000. If there were as many public health nurses as the National Organization for Public Health Nursing recommends (one for every 2,000 or 2,500 population), we should need about 40,000 additional. Also, as sanitation and healthful working conditions come to be taken more for granted as a right of employees, more opportunities for nurses arise in industry. Similarly, higher standards of public service lead to the employment of nurses on trains and airlines. In short, wherever society is dynamic, raising its standards of living and making progress in all kinds of ways, we find the demand for nursing care correspondingly increased.

So it is undoubtedly true that faith in the future of nursing is faith in the future of civilization in general. Of course, if civilization progresses too far, medical science may make its conquest of disease so complete that many fewer nurses will be needed! That is the sort of unemployment, however, that everyone, including nurses, will welcome, but it is so remote a possibility that we can safely ignore it. For a long time to come the growth of the nursing profession will coincide with the growth of civilization.

There is something inspiring about belonging to a profession which is thus closely linked with human progress. There is a zest and sense of adventure in entering a profession which has experienced such phenomenal growth in the present century and is still on the upward march. When we consider that in 1900 there were only 16 graduate and student nurses per 100,000 of population while now there are around 400, it seems almost as if, in the brief course of a half century, we have come out of the dark ages into a new era. But, if we succeed in solving some of our most acute economic problems, the nursing profession may look forward to even greater expansion in the future than it has known in the past.

Incomes in the Nursing Profession

In going into the profession of nursing, you, like other professional people, have probably thought most about what you can do for humanity rather than what you can get out of your career for yourself. At the same time, it is important to have an income which will give you a secure and comfortable living, and you are entirely justified in being concerned about this. You are entitled to ask: What sort of salary will I probably receive, if I become a nurse? And throughout your professional life it is your right and your duty to use your influence and whatever power you possess to see to it that the working conditions and remuneration of nurses are such as will create good morale in the profession.

Now, as for our being able to tell you that you will receive a salary commensurate with your ability, education, and service, we may as well confess at the outset that we can hold forth no such inducement in any profession as long as we live in a man-made world. As long as inequality of the sexes is still the rule and also as long as many women themselves regard their vocation as only a stepping stone to marriage or as a second line of defense in case they fail to get married, we may expect to find women paid at lower rates than men for comparable services. Competition determines this. As long as part of every group of employed women demands only enough pay to get by until marriage, and some, who are partially supported by their parents, require only pin-money, the wage-rates of women in general are bound to be depressed. This is unjust to women who have families to support or who expect to work during an entire lifetime, but not a great deal can be done to correct this injustice, at least until there is more adequate pressure exerted through the creative thinking and work of women at large in every field.

Accepting for the time being this general background of sex inequality, we can speak encouragingly about nursing in merely *relative* terms. In comparison with other vocations for women, nursing rates very favorably. On the basis of studies made by the National Federation of Business and Professional Women's Clubs, the American Journal of Nursing in April, 1938, published the following table of salaries received by women (Table I):

TABLE I: SALARIES RECEIVED BY WOMEN, 1929 AND 1936

	NUMBER REPORTING	MEDIAN SALARY	RANGE OF MIDDLE HALF
In 1929:			
Nurses	509	1,825	1,575–2,180
Librarians	245	1,830	1,395–2,350
Teachers	3,681	1,630	1,240–2,060
Other Professional Workers	5,668	1,715	1,290–2,200
Office Managers	398	1,960	1,610–2,505
Secretaries and Stenographers	2,659	1,620	1,235–1,955
In 1936:			
Nurses	556	1,640	1,235–1,980
Librarians	268	1,485	1,075–1,945
Teachers	3,210	1,375	1,025–1,845
Other Professional Workers	4,692	1,410	1,060–1,880
Office Managers	281	1,470	1,115–1,970
Secretaries and Stenographers	2,604	1,270	920–1,665

These figures represent one of the most prosperous and one of the least prosperous periods in the present century. In each case they probably ran a little too high to be representative of the nation as a whole. Used simply for purposes of comparison, they indicate that nursing stands up well among other women's vocations in remuneration.

Average earnings in various types of nursing, based on reports from a larger number of nurses, will be included among the facts presented in the following section. This information will serve to counteract any misleading impressions obtained from Table I.

Opportunities in Nursing

Graduate registered nurses are found chiefly in four fields: private practice, institutional nursing, public health nursing, and nursing education. In planning your course it is well to decide as soon as possible what type of nursing service you intend to enter. Some familiarity with the different branches of the profession will help you to make up your mind intelligently.

Private Practice. Originally most nurses earned their living through private nursing, since there were few hospitals. A patient with a serious illness had to employ a nurse in his home, or, if he went to a hospital, he had to have a special nurse, for most hospitals employed graduate nurses only in supervisory positions, but depended entirely upon students or upon auxiliary workers for general nursing. At present, however, only about one fourth of all nurses are engaged in private practice. And the decline in the proportion of nurses in private practice will undoubtedly continue for some time until an equilibrium has been reached. Just what this proportion will be will depend upon political and economic factors. Under the best conditions, the amount of private nursing would be stabilized at a very low figure.

Ideally, hospitals should be organized so as to provide highly skilled nursing service for even the most critical cases without its being necessary for the patient to employ a "special" nurse. This will come about as fewer hospitals attempt to conduct schools of nursing, so that hospitals are staffed more and more with graduate nurses instead of students. Such a plan will necessitate somewhat higher charges for hospital services but the average cost per patient will be no greater and probably less, since more efficient use of the time of graduate nurses could be made if they were engaged in general staff duties in a hospital organization instead of wasting time in the care of single patients not critically ill. There would, of course, always be justification for a certain amount of private nursing, but it would be better for the nurse if even these services could be organized through agencies which would maintain a staff of registered nurses on an annual salary basis.

Turning from the ideal to the actual, we can count on the present system of private nursing lasting for many years. For the conscientious and capable nurse who has taken pains to obtain preparation in a wide variety of nursing and who is willing to go out on whatever calls she receives, a career as a private nurse promises a good income and much satisfaction. The disadvantages of irregularity in work and the worries connected with being on one's own are compensated for by the sense of independence, the opportunity to devote more time to the patient, and the great variety of associations and the large number of friendships that grow out of nursing private patients. While the range of incomes is extremely wide (in 1935, when we were still suffering from the depression, the range reported was from $4 to $3,172 for the year), still, this enables the well-prepared and efficient nurse who has good connections to make a higher income than she might as an institutional or public health staff nurse.

The average (median) income of all private nurses in 1936 was $945. The average will necessarily remain quite low as long as there are some nurses (married ones, for example) who are interested in working only part of the time. For those who worked full time (280 or more days a year) the median was $1,260. A survey conducted by the U.S. Department of Commerce in co-operation with the American Nurses' Association in 1941 revealed a median income of $1,168 for private nurses available for employment for at least 48 weeks. The figures just cited do not include the value of meals (if and when received).

Institutional Nursing. The median salary of general staff nurses in hospitals is about the same as the median for private nurses. In 1942 it was $981, not counting maintenance, or $1,200 a year when the value of maintenance is computed. The advantage of employment as a staff nurse is not seen so much in the average salary as in the security and steadiness of employment and the fact that no member of the staff falls below a decent level of living.

In 1941 in small hospitals the median annual income of general staff nurses was $840 plus full maintenance. The median for supervising nurses was $1,020 and for superintendents $1,428, with full maintenance. In 1944 salaries for all institutional nurses ranged from $825 to $7,200 a year, with or without maintenance.

As graduate nurses come to be employed in larger numbers by hospitals, it should be possible to provide careers with opportunity for advancement on any level of nursing. For example, it would be advantageous if certain nurses could set as their objective simply becoming the best possible general staff nurses, with increases in salary as they gained experience and skill. Others who had an aptitude for administration or teaching could go into that type of work. It would then not be necessary for a nurse to advance vertically, so to speak, when she had no inclination for administrative or teaching activities, but she could satisfy her ambitions and receive due reward on a horizontal basis (see Chap. II, p. 20).

Continued growth in the number of institutional nurses will have many important results. One of these should be an increasing recognition of the fact that institutional nursing gives nurses à more independent status economically and professionally.

Public Health Nursing. For those who are qualified and willing to take the additional training required, public health nursing offers an interesting and often inspiring career with relatively high remuneration. And there is every indication that expansion in this field of work will continue for many years.

In 1944 salaries ranged from $840 to $7,200 without maintenance. Median annual salaries for public health nurses in 1942 were as follows:

Staff nurses
 Health departments........................... $1,884
 Non-official agencies......................... 1,608
School nurses..................................... 1,763
Supervisors
 Municipal health departments................. 2,484
 County health departments.................... 1,968
 Non-official agencies......................... 2,004
Directors and associate directors
 Health departments........................... 2,340
 Non-official agencies......................... 2,544

The National Organization for Public Health Nursing recommends that students who plan to become public health nurses should have preparation not only in the more customary services but in the care of patients suffering from tuberculosis, venereal diseases, and acute communicable diseases. The public health nurse should also have had instruction and experience in out-patient clinics, psychiatric nursing, and family health work. Some college study or its equivalent before entering nursing school is advisable in this as in all fields. For the public health nurse who takes a position in which she has to work alone, the

National Organization for Public Health Nursing recommends a year of post-graduate study and at least one year of experience under supervision in a public health nursing service which emphasizes family health. For a supervisor or director it is recommended that the nurse have a college education, special preparation in public health nursing, advanced work in education or the theory and practice of supervision, and two or more years experience in public health nursing.

Public health nursing, which has been in existence in this country for more than a half century, was originally conducted for the most part by private charitable agencies. In recent decades, however, the trend has been strongly in the direction of more governmental agencies and fewer private ones. Now three-fourths of all public health nursing is governmental. The lively public interest in health and the increasing pressure upon the federal government to insure adequate medical care for low-income groups bid fair to increase still further the number and proportion of government public health nurses. The Social Security Act and the National Health Act are only beginnings.

When H. G. Wells published his conception of The Rights of Man some years ago, the most significant thing about his statement was the inclusion of the *right to health*. As we come to recognize generally that all men are entitled to good medical and nursing care simply by virtue of the fact that they are human beings, the government is virtually certain to be a major factor in implementing such a right, seeing to it that it is more than a pious phrase. This will probably mean not only many additional public health nurses but also large numbers of general staff nurses in the employ of the government.

Federal Government Services. While we are talking about the part which the government is playing and will play in providing nursing care for certain sections of the population, it must not be forgotten that the Federal Government employs nurses in practically all fields of work. Increasingly it has developed institutional, public health, nursing education and military services. The specific Federal agencies employing the largest number of nurses are the Army Nurse Corps, the Navy Nurse Corps, the U. S. Public Health Service (operating often through state and local agencies), the Office of Indian Affairs, and the U.S.

Veterans' Administration. Salaries of nurses in these and other Federal nursing services are variable but an index of them is found in the initial salaries of nurses in the Army and Navy. These salaries in 1945 were $1800 per year plus subsistence and allowances amounting to about $800, or a total of approximately $2600. For more detailed information the student may consult *Facts about Nursing* and *Nursing, a Profession for College Women* published by The Nursing Information Bureau.

Industrial Nursing. Nurses in the employ of industrial and commercial concerns have usually been classified as public health nurses, but a few words may be added here regarding this phase of nursing. Increasing numbers of nurses are being employed in industry not only because under workmen's compensation laws it pays the employer to maintain a low sickness and accident rate but also because many employers have a genuine concern for the well-being of their employees. A well-trained and socially conscious nurse in an industrial position can make excellent contributions to public health education through contacts with workers and their families.

Nursing Education. One field in which the demand has exceeded the supply of qualified persons is that of teaching. Especially in recent years when standards of nursing education have been raised, it has been difficult to find nurses with the additional education required to fill administrative and teaching positions. Nursing schools which are conducted by hospitals mainly as a means of obtaining cheap nursing services have been steadily losing ground and will eventually have to be abandoned or converted into genuine educational institutions. Since nursing organizations have set standards of preparation comparable with those of other college courses and are enforcing these standards by means of accrediting, there is an increased demand for nurses who desire to specialize in nursing education and have been willing to take the time and make the effort which preparation for teaching and administration requires. Salaries are comparable to those of women teachers in high schools and colleges. In 1944 they ranged from $825 to $7,200 a year, with or without maintenance.

In order to become a member of the staff of a school of nursing, the student should plan to take a college course with a major in nursing education (leading to at least a bachelor's degree), in addition to the usual professional preparation for nursing. Advanced work in those subjects in which the nurse may want to specialize should also be taken. Above all, in a changing world, it is important for nursing educators to have a liberal education so that the schools which they conduct will prepare nurses to deal intelligently with the social, political, and economic conditions upon which the health of the public depends as much as it does upon the science and art of nursing itself. Especially with the recent emphasis upon the preventive aspects of medicine and nursing, schools of nursing must prepare nurses who will reduce disease by enlightening the public rather than merely care for patients at the bedside. In a certain sense every nurse in the future will be an educator, whether she specializes in education or not.

Various Specializations. If space permitted, we might go into detail about many specialized opportunities for nurses. All that we can do, however, is to mention some of these and suggest that students obtain literature from their advisers and occupational counselors or from national nursing organizations and read this through before making a final decision regarding the particular field of nursing into which they will go.

It has sometimes been difficult to find sufficient nurses specially prepared for pediatrics, obstetrics, communicable diseases (including tuberculosis), orthopedics, psychiatry, and outpatient services. There are opportunities also for nurse anesthetists, x-ray technicians, office nurses, nursing school librarians, medical record librarians, physical therapists, and occupational therapists. In addition to administrative work in hospitals and public health services, there are a few executive positions with state boards of nurse examiners and with nursing organizations.

Men Nurses. The general public rarely thinks of men in the nursing profession, but there are two fields in which there is a demand for a considerable number of men—psychiatric and urologic nursing. Some opportunities are also opening up in pediatrics, and a limited number of competent men nurses can expect fairly steady employment as private nurses, with remuneration somewhat higher than that received by women. Just prior to our entrance into the second World War there were about 8,000 men nurses in this country. In 1943 there were 76 schools which accepted both men and women students, and four which accepted men only.

Your Career

From what you have read in this chapter and the introduction you can perhaps appreciate more fully than previously the remarkable character and scope of the profession which you are entering. Professions usually require hundreds of years in which to develop but the present century has seen two, in which women play predominant parts, rise to maturity in an incredibly short time—social work and nursing. The first steps in making nursing a profession in the United States were taken as far back as 1873, when several hospitals founded schools with formal training programs. Only in the period following the first World War did nursing really establish itself as a profession, however. Registered nurses increased from 66,000 in 1918 to about a third of a million at present. Thus, you have the privilege of entering upon your career just at the time when nursing is attaining its maturity.

We can reaffirm, therefore, that nursing offers you an opportunity to make your future a good and highly useful one. This is true regardless of whether it becomes for you a life-time and full-time career or whether marriage intervenes to prevent this. Something will be said later about the possibility of women having careers outside the home and at the same time rearing families. Whether you believe that such a combination of functions is practicable or not, nursing has this advantage, as compared with many other types of training for women, that it will always be a practical possession in any kind of life. The economic waste of training women for careers only to have them abandon them as soon as possible after marriage is in general appalling. Yet, when a graduate nurse gives up her career, her preparation still remains of great practical value to her, for example, in the care of her children. Also, as a member in the Reserve of the American Red Cross Nursing Service, she can stand ready to serve the nation in time of disaster or national emergency. And she can also be an educational and political force for enlightenment and health in her community. In a certain sense, then, no nurse can ever abandon her career completely.

We have talked in this chapter about the opportunities which nursing offers for you. Let us now consider, in what follows, the abilities and qualities that are required in one who hopes to become a nurse. What makes a good nurse? What adjustments must a student expect to make in preparing for the nursing profession?

Study Questions

1. What evidence can you give to indicate that the nursing profession is on an ascending curve of development?

2. Contrast ideal with actual employment conditions in nursing, as they have existed in the past.

3. Explain how the purchasing power of the public affects the service of the nurse to society.

4. In what ways has government fostered the extension and improvement of nursing service?

Questions for Thought and Discussion

1. Think back to the period of your life before you entered the school of nursing; try to recollect the factors which influenced you to choose nursing as a career. List these factors for your own use.

2. Has your concept of nursing as a career changed or been enlarged since you began your professional studies? Explain your present reasons for wanting to become a nurse.

3. Indicate some of the ways in which your future and that of the profession of nursing are dependent upon human progress itself.

4. What public health nursing agencies exist in your community? County? State? What is the chief function of each of these agencies?

5. Why do we refer to plans such as those of group hospitalization as being typically democratic in character?

6. Some doctors have opposed the establishment of group health plans. Discuss the question: Will group health plans put private physicians out of practice?

7. What opportunities are there in your community for participation in group hospitalization plans? In other health insurance plans?

8. Discuss the statement: ". . . if civilization progresses too far, medical science may make its conquest of disease so complete that many fewer nurses will be needed!"

9. What is your reaction to this remark made by a nurse student: "I think I'll be a general duty nurse when I graduate; I'd like to live in the nurses' residence and have no responsibilities for rent, light, and so forth."

10. Suggest some ways in which the married nurse may render nursing service in her home and in the community.

Books to Read

Occupational Literature

Most of the facts presented in this chapter have been derived from publications which you may be interested in reading yourself. They can be found in libraries and in school offices or counseling bureaus, or you may prefer to write and obtain some of the literature from the Nursing Information Bureau of the American Nurses' Association, New York City. The exact address you can always learn by inquiring at your school of nursing office and by consulting the official directory in the American Journal of Nursing. A few of the titles are the following:

Books

Nursing as a Profession by Esther Lucille Brown (published by Russell Sage Foundation, New York, 2nd Ed., 1940).

A Short History of Nursing by Lavinia L. Dock, R.N., and Isabel M. Stewart, R.N. (published by Putnam's, New York, 1938).

A Short Life of Florence Nightingale by Rosalind Nash (published by Macmillan Co., New York, 1926).

Biographical Sketches of American Nurses (booklets and individual sketches, published by the National League of Nursing Education, New York).

Penny Marsh, Public Health Nurse, by Dorothy Deming, R.N. (published by Dodd, Mead Co., New York, 1938).

Edith Cavell, by Helen Judson (published by Macmillan Co., New York, 1941).

Your Career in Nursing by Cecilia L. Schulz, R.N. (published by Whittlesey House, 1941).

Pamphlets

Publications of the Nursing Information Bureau of the American Nurses' Association and the National League of Nursing Education, New York:

Facts about Nursing. 25 cents.
Nursing and How to Prepare for It. Free.
Nursing and the Registered Professional Nurse. 10 cents.
Nursing — A Profession for College Women. 25 cents.
The ANA and You. Free.
Opportunities in Nursing. Free.

Publications of the National Organization for Public Health Nursing, New York:

Your Career—Will it be Public Health Nursing? Free.
How to Enter the Field of Public Health Nursing. Free.
The Nurse in the Industrial Health Program. Free.

Publications of the American National Red Cross, Washington, D. C.:·

American Red Cross Nursing Service. Free.
Facts. Free.

Publications of U.S. Department of Labor Women's Bureau, Washington, D. C:

Professional Nurses (Bulletin 203 No. 3). Free.

Publication of the Public Affairs Committee, Inc., New York:

Better Nursing for America by Beulah Amidon
(Public Affairs Pamphlet, No. 60) 10 cents.

Magazines

(The student should early form the habit of keeping up with professional journals in her field, even before she has had enough preparation to comprehend all the articles appearing in them.)

American Journal of Nursing
Public Health Nursing
International Nursing Review

II

What Makes a Good Nurse

A STUDENT, at the beginning of her program in nursing, is interested in knowing "what makes a good nurse." She is concerned to see a total, though brief, picture of what lies ahead of her, both as a student and as a graduate. She wishes to give careful consideration to the problems which she will face.

It is not easy to discuss these problems directly. There is a story in Greek mythology, however, which may give us a cue as to how to approach them. It is the well-known tale of how Perseus killed Medusa, the Fury with snaky locks. The difficulty in killing Medusa was that she turned to stone anyone who gazed at her. Thus had many heroes perished who, before Perseus, attempted the feat. Perseus, however, invented a different technic of approach by using his brightly polished shield as a mirror. In it he could see Medusa and aim his blow at her without being turned to stone.

In this chapter we shall imitate Perseus' method of approach. Carrying the shield of our profession so brightly polished that we can see our problems in it, and in it only, we shall use it as a guide in our attack. Like Perseus, we shall advance upon our difficulties circuitously by considering first a general formula for satisfactory attainment in nursing.

In choosing a profession, one of the most important considerations is to obtain ultimate satisfaction in one's own work. But to attain this we must do work that is socially significant, work that enhances the physical, mental, spiritual welfare of human beings. The work must bring a needed service to society. It must be worthwhile. In other words, it must fit into the pattern which is the ideal of our profession.

Attainment is not the result of a single factor but depends upon a number of related factors, of which three are essential: first, the endowment one brings to the task of nursing; second, the preparation one achieves for the task; and, third, the specific task within the field of nursing one selects eventually as her very own. Before discussing these essentials, let us examine some criteria for measuring vocational satisfaction in nursing.

Criteria of Success

There are two types of criteria, which may be called the *vertical* and the *horizontal*. In the past we have been accustomed to use as a criterion of successful attainment in nursing the vertical measuring rod. This gauge, which is individualistic in character, indicated a person's status on an ascending, descending scale. Promotion of a nurse in an institution, for example, was from staff nurse to head nurse, from head nurse to supervisor, from supervisor to instructor, from instructor to assistant director, and from assistant director to director. Her satisfaction tended to depend upon her promotion from one type of activity to another, and the higher the level attained the greater the nurse's satisfaction. We are all elated when a staff nurse is promoted to the position of head nurse. But the future points to a different scale of valuation—a change from the vertical to the horizontal scale. On the basis of the latter, advancement may occur without the necessity of giving up the type of nursing service which one prefers. A few agencies already recognize progressive improvement in quality of "bedside" nursing by increases in salary for the staff nurse. Or, a nurse who wants to do some administrative work may with proper promotions remain as an experienced and excellent head nurse. An example of this is found in English hospitals where ward sisters (head nurses) take pride in maintaining the same position for life.

The two methods of rating progress are indicated in the following graph:

A. Vertical Progress	B. Horizontal Progress
Director	Inexperienced→Experienced
↑	
Assistant Director	Inexperienced→Experienced
↑	
Instructor	Inexperienced→Experienced
↑	
Supervisor	Inexperienced→Experienced
↑	
Head Nurse	Inexperienced→Experienced
↑	
Staff Nurse	Inexperienced→Experienced

The criterion of success, then, will be increased competence in the field selected. With this broader conception of success in mind, let us turn now to a consideration of the three factors which contribute to a satisfying career as a nurse.

Factors Contributing to Success and Satisfaction

Just as in the laboratory we may select and combine elements to secure a desired result and control these in such a way as to be sure of the final product, so in nursing we may achieve satisfaction and successful service to the community by a proper combination of personal, educational, and vocational factors. We are to discuss, then, the elements in the formula:

Capacity + Preparation + Choice of Work ——→ Satisfaction.

Individual Capacity

The first and most important element in our formula will be found in ourselves. What we are and what we bring to nursing determine in large measure the success and satisfaction we achieve in it. The whole process starts with us and returns to us.

There are two ways of finding out whether or not we should be in nursing. One of these is the "trial and error," or "trial and success" method. The other may be called, for lack of a better term, the scientific method. Under the former, the most commonly used method in the past, a student tries nursing. If she succeeds, well and good. If not, well, but not so good. We all know people who have taken nursing courses and succeeded in outstanding fashion. We know others who have tried nursing and failed. In the scientific method, counseling or guidance services assist the student in evaluating her abilities and aptitudes for specific fields of work, including that of nursing. This counseling should be had preferably before a student enters a nursing school but may be sought afterward if desired. In either case, the combination of factors that make her what she is will form the determinants of success and satisfaction in her chosen field, in so far as the student as an individual is concerned.

Let us assume that a student will use the scientific method for evaluating her fitness for nursing. There is scarcely anything about one, from hairdress to choice of profession, which a counseling service may not study and upon which it may not advise. From the list of possible essentials, let us consider a number of these under two headings which we shall call *aptitude for nursing* and *ability for nursing*.

Aptitude. Under the head of aptitude, a vocational counselor might well consider *temperament, adjustment,* and *personality*. These often form the key to one's entire life pattern. They hold first rank for all of us in defining immediate and ultimate success, on either a vertical or horizontal scale. We have all seen the nurse who is adequate in any emergency. Perhaps, we have seen, also, one who goes to pieces under strain. We all know the person of excellent adjustment: one whose personal life is without undue conflict, whose family relationships are happy, and who forms a pleasant member of her social group. She is likely to have a pleasing and interesting personality, to make and keep friends easily, and to be well liked by all with whom she comes in contact. Such a person tends to make a well-adjusted and contented nurse.

Another factor that will claim the attention of a counselor is that of *motivation*, your reason for entering the profession of nursing. The higher the motivation you have for entering the profession and for going into any specific work within it, the greater, other things being equal, will be your satisfaction in the field. Is a student entering nursing because she knows something of the service it offers people and because she wishes to be prepared to render that service? If so, she is apt to be satisfied. Is she entering because there is no other opening, or possibly because the uniform appeals to her? Her chances of satisfaction are not so high. There comes to mind a student whose desire to enter nursing dated back to her childhood days when she saw an injured mother go without much-needed nursing care. From this experience grew her resolve to be prepared when she grew up to give that care to others who might need it. Coupled closely to motivation as a factor in success and satisfaction is *interest* in the work you are doing. Patients will often remark upon the care given them by an interested nurse even though the care may be inferior in quality.

Less easily judged in vocational counseling is that personality trait known as *social sensitivity*. Much like personal sympathy, it goes beyond the immediate situation, impelling one to action in promotion of desirable conditions. The socially sensitive student, for example, is concerned not only to recognize symptoms and give treatment, but to investigate and use her influence for correcting the social conditions which give rise to the condition. Dr. Hilda Taba cites an example of a child suffering from malnutrition.* The socially sensitive nurse is one who not only wishes to care for the child and treat it well but who is concerned also to see that the conditions which originally led to malnutrition are corrected.

Ability. Better understood than the foregoing aptitudes are the more obvious grades of *physical* and *mental ability* required for nursing work. There is little use trying to do what one has really not the power and strength to do.

In considering one's ability from a physical point of view, we think primarily of health. We want to have health in the positive sense of the word, not a mere absence of illness. This positive health will stand us in good stead when days of overwork occur and unforeseen emergencies tax us as they will and must. Perhaps as physical concomitants might be mentioned such matters as appearance and speech. They are considered important enough by some counseling agencies to merit special consultant services. What patient has not been cheered by the presence of an attractive, well-groomed nurse? What one has not been comforted and soothed by the well-modulated voice of an understanding nurse?

So far as mental ability is concerned, definite measurements are available to gauge mental ability to handle a nursing curriculum. Such measurements may be helpful as a warning sign to avoid what might be a basic cause of dissatisfaction in nursing. A student who comes into nursing only to find that her mental equipment will function better in some other field should seek that field immediately rather than run the chance of permanent dissatisfaction.

Preparation

Equal in importance to individual capacity is the second element, preparation. While much of the actual control of a student's preparation lies outside her own immediate province,

* Taba, Hilda, "Social Sensitivity—Its Implications for Nursing," The Minnesota Registered Nurse, December, 1940, pp. 8–9.

nevertheless she should be aware of the elements in her program which will contribute to a successful career. Not infrequently students themselves have been responsible for improvements in their preparation. An illustration of this may be cited. A group of students requested the privilege of better experience in the care of the normal child. This request was referred to the curriculum committee of the faculty and thence to the faculty itself. It received favorable action. Initiation of the effort to improve this experience came from the students themselves. If students are endowed with proper personality (as used here), most schools of nursing will, we believe, welcome their suggestions and cooperation in procuring the best possible preparation for nursing. Another example may not be amiss. Here some students asked if a member of the faculty might not have more time for counseling them about their problems. This request was appreciated and met as the situation allowed.

There are two approaches to the problem of preparing for nursing, an earlier and a more modern approach. In a consideration of the *earlier*, it is well to remember that nursing education is functional in character. Nurses learn by doing. They learn to nurse by nursing. The learning process takes place in large measure in actual nursing situations. This is why even a comparatively planless preparation of students in nursing is often successful. If the student happens to be in a good learning situation, if she is in a school with access to many types of patients in adequate numbers, and if the teaching personnel is good, the chances are that the student will receive an adequate preparation. Indeed, it may even be excellent. On the other hand, her preparation under such a system may be very limited. For example, her experience may include only the care of medical and surgical patients. Under this planless system, chance plays too important a role in a nurse's preparation.

In the *modern approach*, the preparation of the student is more planful. Schools are able to put into operation programs that are increasingly well systematized. Of the many important phases of a modern planful preparation, let us select four factors for brief consideration. The first of these has to do with the situation, the second with the faculty, the third with the curriculum, and the fourth with the student.

In a well-planned scheme, the *situation* in which students study nursing should provide a satisfactory learning laboratory. Such a program should, we assume, facilitate learning. It should be built primarily to meet the needs of students. It should be satisfactory in the following respects: adequate facilities for learning nursing, a fair balance between work and play, and desirable living conditions allowing a wholesome social life. Adequate facilities imply among other things adequate numbers of patients and a library. The American Red Cross Nursing Service requires that a nurse's preparation be secured in a situation involving a minimum daily average of fifty patients. Many smaller schools meet this requirement through affiliation by sending their students to a larger school for a portion of their experience.

Balance between work and play is often determined by the functional character of a nurse's preparation. Recognition of the value of her practice in an actual nursing situation may bring in its train such causes of dissatisfaction as long hours, the care of too many patients to do satisfactory work, and the too extended performance of non-nursing duties. An extreme example of the latter may be seen in the following instance. An acquaintance many years ago visited a school of nursing. The head of the school displayed the garden surrounding the hospital and commented that each student nurse spent a definite period of time working in the garden, adding, "You see, we stress most the practical." Fortunately, we no longer find such extreme instances but examples illustrative of the subordination of student needs are familiar to all of us. Of course, it may have been the maid's fault when, on another occasion, a nurse, coming into a large but darkened and dusty living room of a nurses' residence, asked the maid if she had dusted the living room, and got the response, "No, wuz you goin' to use it?"

Our second factor in good preparation is the *faculty*. The ideal faculty is interested in the student, understands her problems, is neither too busy nor too aloof to consider them with her. We think of a student who found at the last moment that her father could not provide the necessary funds for payment of her living expenses during the period when this was required. Upon consideration of her case, a scholarship was secured for her. In another, but similar, case an instructor actually took the student into her own home. While scholarships or homes may not always be available, ideally there will always be a faculty alert to the needs of students, a faculty to whom the students will feel free to come for guidance. The ideal faculty will be qualified and competent to provide for the student a high quality of teaching and supervision. It will, in so far as it is humanly possible, be accurate in rating the student's class work and practice. It will further contribute to such faculty-student relationships as to make student life both pleasant and stimulating.

The *curriculum* is the instrument through which you get on with the job of learning nursing. It should provide teaching and experience in all important basic nursing services if you are to be adequately prepared to make suitable workers for the jobs you will eventually hold. It is this instrument that gives you the necessary knowledge for the job. It may not fit you for particular positions but it should train you in such basic fields as medical, surgical, pediatric, obstetric, psychiatric, and tuberculosis nursing.

Important as the faculty and curriculum are, the *student's contribution* is paramount. Ultimately it is she who does the really important part of preparing herself for the work, for only that knowledge is really useful which is so thoroughly absorbed that it enters into one's own personality and becomes a vital part of it. The school of nursing may search the world over for the effective in training, but the student must bring a great part of the effectiveness in herself. The school may provide the tools of preparation—the situation, the faculty, and the curriculum—but only the student can utilize them to the fullest measure.

Choice of Work

We have been speaking thus far of the first two elements in our formula, individual capacity and preparation. Coordinate in value with them is the third element, right choice of work. Even as a young student you will be giving serious thought to the choice of work which you will eventually make.

Choice of work may be made in one of two ways, the subjective or the objective. In the past, the tendency was for nurses to make this selection subjectively. A nurse's choice depended almost entirely on her personal preference in the matter, and was heavily weighted with subjective considerations. A nurse would sample various fields of work or specific jobs and if she liked the work would stay in it. If, however, her occupational choice proved to be a mistake, either through dislike of the work, or lack of success in it, she would change her field of endeavor. In more recent years, nurses, like other workers, have tended more and more to make their selection of work as far as possible objectively. They still rely upon their personal preferences, but in addition they also utilize scientific methods of guidance as aids in the selection. These newer methods take account of the individual's interests as well as aptitudes, abilities, and preparation. They are not infallible guides to a choice of work, but studies of comparable groups show a far higher percentage of advised than of unadvised persons planning to follow the work of their choice.*

Among the other matters which a guidance service will consider are actual preference, employer, and conditions of work. A good counselor will wish to know whether you are really in a position to choose. Perhaps personal or family situations, or a strong sense of duty, may compel you to select a certain kind of position in a special place and at a particular salary, in preference to another more desirable opportunity. Again, a counselor will usually feel that, other things being equal, it is wise to select work in which the employer-employee relationships are pleasant. Granted that one does not work for praise alone, all of us tend to do better work under approval than under disapproval. In addition, a counselor will give special consideration to what may be termed "conditions of work." Her attention in this connection will be centered upon matters such as the nature of the work, opportunities for advancement, and factors involved in salary, hours of work, and tenure. She will probably rank as the most important of these the type or nature of the work to be chosen. She will feel that

* An example of this is cited in R. Hoppock's and C. Odom's article "Job Satisfaction" in *Occupations*, 19:24–28. In a comparison of two groups of boys it was found five years later that 72 per cent of the advised boys were planning to follow their present work whereas 65 per cent of the unadvised ones hoped to change their work.

the work should have an appeal to you, that it should seem important to you, that it should be of a kind in which you can feel a creative joy and in which the environment is pleasing and satisfying. She will stress the need of considering opportunities for advancement. In fact, she may emphasize the need of selecting every job on the basis of its value as a preparation for the next job. She will be concerned that the remuneration shall be commensurate with that of workers in other fields for comparable work, though in a profession this will never be her primary consideration. In fact, for first positions she will consider salary of far less importance than the nature of the work. She will advise consideration of work that does not entail hours that are too long or too strenuous for healthful living. She will not be unmindful of a healthful social environment. Last, but not least, she will advise a position in which it is possible to build up a fair degree of security.

Considering, then, yourself and your preparation and making use of whatever services you can, in the last analysis it must fall to you as an individual to make the choice of the field in which you will work. You alone can do this. Each individual must select her own niche. As William James said, "Vocational biographies will never be written in advance." Fortunately, choice of work may be, and usually is, a dynamic, continuous process. It need never be entirely settled. For in the process of arriving at our goals of satisfactory service on either a vertical or a horizontal basis, we are constantly vouchsafed the privilege and the need of renewal of choice. Attainment, success, satisfaction; these are the result of a whole network of factors. What we are; what preparation we acquire; what choice of work we make;—the combination of all these, together with their various concomitants, determines the service we will render, the social values we will contribute, and finally, the satisfaction we ourselves will derive from our work. It was William James, too, who said that contentment equals the ratio between pretension and attainment. You may have seen the picture of a captain, a cook, and a first mate. The captain is happy. He wanted to be a captain. He prepared to be a captain. He is a captain. Attainment is equal to pretension. The cook is beamingly happy. He wanted to be a cook. He is a cook. He wouldn't be anything else in the world. The first mate is a fine man. You think you see this in his face. But he wanted to be a captain and didn't make it.

These are the two ways, the vertical and the horizontal. In the first, the past American way, pretension or ambition has run high. One could only succeed by climbing up. In the second, our proposed newer way, we change the pretension and achieve satisfaction by extending our service horizontally in a chosen field of work. What we set ourselves to do we must attain, if we are to be happy. But if we start with a mistaken set, it is better to change the set and so attain happiness than to live the dissatisfied life of the first mate. As the poet said,

"Tis the set of the sails and not the gales
That determines the way they go."

In any case, we are prepared now to make our choices with some knowledge of the general conditions that determine success and satisfaction in nursing. Let us next proceed to something a little more specific—the adjustments that the student may expect to make in the first part of her career as a student.

Study Questions

1. Describe two methods of evaluating success in nursing.
2. What three factors are essential to attainment in nursing?
3. How may a prospective student find out whether she should enter the basic professional program in nursing?

Questions for Thought and Discussion

1. Why is it better use of human resources to give salary and rank promotion within each type of nursing service, rather than to compel nurses to "advance themselves" by moving from one type of service to another, for example, from teaching to administration?
2. Why is it important for a student to examine the educational offerings of the school in which she wishes to enroll? in which she is enrolled?
3. Discuss the statement: "If you work hard enough and long enough at any given task, success is bound to reward your effort."

4. Make a list of the types of nursing service which appeal to you as possible careers.

5. List the personal and professional qualifications which you think would be required for success in the jobs listed in number 4 above.

6. Could you meet these requirements? If not, how would you plan to develop the necessary qualifications?

Books to Read

Cabot, Richard Clarke: *Meaning of Right and Wrong.* Rev. Ed. New York. Macmillan. 1936.

Fosdick, Harry Emerson: *Twelve Tests of Character.* New York. Association Press. 1923.

Fosdick, Harry Emerson: *On Being a Real Person.* New York. Harper & Bros. 1943.

Nightingale, Florence: *Talks to Pupils: A Selection of Addresses to Probationers and Nurses.* New York. Macmillan. 1914.

Nightingale, Florence: *Notes on Nursing.* New York. Appleton. 1860.

Sutherland, Dorothy Gertrude: *Do You Want to Be a Nurse?* New York. Doubleday, Doran. 1942.

Triggs, Frances Oralind: *Counseling in Schools of Nursing.* Philadelphia. Saunders. 1945.

III

Initial Adjustments

During recent decades there has been much talk about adjustment—adjustment of younger people to school environment, adjustment of adults to society, and adjustment of those whose life work is devoted to a profession or to various institutions. Psychiatrists, and personnel counselors especially, have made much of this concept, for they have been chiefly concerned with helping the individual to get along well and to achieve success with a minimum of friction. They are right, therefore, in emphasizing adjustment, since everyone needs to learn this art of fitting in.

The Meaning of Adaptation. But, before we discuss some of the adjustments that a nurse must make, let us get clear in our minds the limitations of any narrow interpretation of this "adjustment outlook" on life. In order to see that "fitting in" is only the first step in a worthwhile life, let us ask whether some of the great benefactors of mankind have been well adjusted individuals. Did Socrates, Jesus, Savonarola, Galileo, Lincoln, and Florence Nightingale adapt themselves to the society of their day? Did they fit in? Were they so well adjusted that they caused no trouble for the people or institutions with which they came in contact? Was the entire life of each nothing but smooth sailing? Obviously not, since Socrates and Jesus were condemned to death, Savonarola was mobbed, Galileo came close to losing his life, Lincoln was assassinated, and Florence Nightingale had to struggle against the conservatism and lack of vision of her contemporaries. No one would think of judging them by the standard of whether they adjusted themselves to their environment. Rather, we glorify them for opposing evil institutions and for creating new and better ones. Far from adapting themselves to their environment, they strove to reform their environment and to fit it to the dream of a better world that was within them. It was Florence Nightingale who said, "I can mould circumstances, not circumstances me."

It would thus be ludicrous, if not indeed blasphemous, to ask of any of our great men and women: Did they adjust themselves well? How much progress would the world make if everyone adjusted himself perfectly to existing institutions? Very little indeed. Yet everywhere today we hear the gospel of "adjustment" preached, and even in this book we find ourselves discussing the subject. This certainly may seem inconsistent, but actually it is not, because both adjustment and non-adjustment have a proper place in the scheme of life. The reformers mentioned above illustrate the value of non-adjustment in achieving progress. On the other hand, the great institutions of our twentieth-century civilization illustrate the value of adjustment, for their achievements depend on the cooperation of the people who compose them. After all, even the staunchest rebels and reformers have had to begin their careers by conforming to the rules of institutions in which they worked. They would not have commanded a hearing had they not at first fitted into the existing order sufficiently to rise to positions of influence. Chronic maladjustment and inability to cooperate are not signs of originality and genius nor do they give promise of future creative work.

Another way of reconciling a philosophy of adjustment with a philosophy of social progress is to think of adjustment as a two-way process which consists not only in a modification of the individual so that he may work cooperatively with others but also in a modification of institutions by individuals. Adaptation, for an intelligent animal like man, means not merely adapting himself to his environment but adapting the environment to himself. Adjustment means the "give-and-take" that results in harmonious relations in the long run, though not always in the short run.

All of which is simply by way of placing in its proper perspective the advice to be given in the following pages. We do not want to appear to be initiating you into an army to do what you are told as a matter of discipline, without ever a question or a doubt. As will be shown in a subsequent chapter, we are primarily interested in seeing the nursing profession composed of intelligent, enlightened, socially minded persons, who are capable of doing original and constructive thinking about social institutions, including their own profession But no one is competent to judge the workings of an institution or to suggest changes in it until she has first sincerely tried to live up to its rules and to understand their purpose. A critic is more likely to command attention if she has manifested an ability to submit cheerfully and cooperatively in a situation before beginning to propose changes.

Some General Rules for Intelligent Adjustment

The following suggestions may be of help in making your first adjustments to school and hospital while at the same time not surrendering completely your intelligence:

1. Realize that in a nursing (or medical) organization strict observance of rules by everyone is of the utmost importance. It may be a matter of life or death.
2. It takes time to appreciate the reason for some regulations. Requirements which may seem petty to you now will impress you later as being highly important in maintaining efficient hospital and nursing service.
3. Institutions are not perfect and many of them suffer from "cultural lag," that is, some customs persist long after they have lost their usefulness (and some may never have had any rational justification in the first place!). You may, therefore, be quite right in thinking that some rules are foolish. But even in these cases it is best to suspend final judgment until you have had more experience. In the meantime show a cooperative spirit and good sportsmanship by conforming cheerfully. Later, when you have attained a place in an organization where you can initiate reforms, then you may become aggressively critical.
4. In case a regulation is so obviously unreasonable and out of touch with reality that there is general dissatisfaction with it, do not just "gripe" about it privately but take steps to have it discussed by your student organization. Representatives may then confer with the proper author-

ities. If there is no student organization to handle such matters, take steps in cooperation with the proper authorities to form such an organization. Most good schools of nursing now have some form of student government.

5. Do not request special privileges for yourself or make an exception of yourself. If you are tempted to do this, ask yourself the simple question: "What if everybody should do as I am doing? What sort of school or hospital would this be if everyone did as I am about to do?"

6. Try to understand and appreciate some of the factors leading to nursing "lag." This lag might be defined as the gap between theory and practice. It is the difference between what you are taught and what you may at times see practiced in the care of patients. Probably in no sphere of activity will your ideals and your practices always be commensurate. While the hospital makes every attempt to ensure safe and really fine care for all patients, there will doubtless be times of emergency or of pressure of work when it will be impossible to do as much as you would like in the time allotted. In situations such as these you will avoid a great deal of unhappiness if you have an understanding of the need for the shortcuts, and if you have the judgment of the nurse in charge as to what cuts may be made safely.

With these admonitions in mind, let us now make a brief survey of some of the things that are expected of students and nurses in most institutions.

Adult Responsibilities

When you take up nursing you are expected to have an adult attitude toward life. Young people going to college are often told that they must look upon their program of study as equivalent to the work of an adult. For one thing, they are expected to carry about fifteen hours of class per week and to study approximately thirty hours (two hours for each hour of class), making a total of forty-five hours. This is about what would be expected in a full-time working week. For many students such a program represents their first adult job, though the hours may not be as regular as in other jobs. Furthermore, students must, in most cases, assume full responsibility for doing their work satisfactorily and for living a well-rounded life. The school provides conditions conducive to study and wholesome living, together with all sorts of aids and guidance for the student, but in the last analysis it is the individual who must decide whether she will "take it or leave it." There is no attempt at pampering, or coddling, and the student must stand on her own two feet. As students in nursing, you are accepted as adults and are expected to bear the responsibilities of maturity. What, then, are some of the implications of this new status for you as an adult individual?

Budget of Time. One of the most important implications under this new status is that you will require some sort of plan to achieve any degree of effectiveness. No longer can you feel free to do things just as they come up. You must learn to schedule your activities somewhat in advance or else find that many worthwhile phases of living will escape you. Of course, some sort of plan may eventually evolve spontaneously out of your experience, but it will help greatly if you will take those seven days (each with its twenty-four hours) at your disposal, and deliberately budget the time for each. Allow what you need for sleep, for meals, for "on duty," for class, for study, for recreation, and you will be surprised how much more you can do with allotted time than would be possible without such a prearranged plan.

As a special example of the need for planning let us consider the matter of organizing your study activity. A student is wise if she recognizes from the outset that everything she learns will find a useful application in her future work. Every class period, as well as the preparation for it, is absolutely indispensable. Only if a definite study plan is strictly adhered to will the full value of class work be realized; bluffing or cramming will only defeat you in the long run.

In the matter of organizing such a study plan some faculty member will always be ready to offer you helpful advice. Such a plan must take into consideration such things as: (1) the development of good study habits; (2) proper spacing of class and study periods, including the placing of study periods after class hours; (3) allowance of extra time for subjects which offer greater difficulty. Furthermore, the plan must also provide some means for testing your accomplishments in your studies. It should, however, be sufficiently flexible so that if you should wish to employ a regular study evening for some recreational activity, you could, without upsetting your schedule, devote to studying an evening usually given over to recreation. Finally, for effective studying one needs a comfortable place (but not so comfortable as to induce drowsiness!).

No plan, of course, works perfectly, but one must realize the fundamental fact that any plan is much better than no plan. Just as in making a dress you rely upon a pattern, or in erecting a house you depend upon a blueprint, so in building a professional career why not dispose planfully the most precious item— your time?

Budget of Money. You are fortunate if from childhood you have been accustomed to living within a budget. The amount of money you will need depends upon the type of curriculum you are carrying, a "degree" or a "diploma" program, since the cost of the former will be greater than of the latter. While the expense for the student during pre-nursing and post-nursing periods is usually comparable to that of other college students, the expense during the actual nursing period (clinical experience) is, in most places, much less. But whatever the cost of a program may be, the important thing for most of us is, (1) to set up some sort of workable budget which allows for such anticipated expenditures as books, tuition, maintenance, clothing, recreation, and so forth, and then (2) to try to live within that budget, no matter how small it is. The wise individual will also save some small portion of her allowance. The items which trouble most students are clothing, food, and recreation, with clothing topping the list.

Clothing. Probably none of us uses perfect judgment and taste in the matter of clothes. A few simple maxims, if followed, would, however, spare us much financial and personal embarrassment. You can, for example, wear but one dress at a time. Then why have many? Or, "Be not the first by whom the new is tried, nor yet the last to lay the old aside." One of the best dressed young women we know had in three years only one suit (with separate blouses), two dinner and two evening dresses in addition to a coverall coat which she wore for several years. These few outfits were all of the same color so that accessories for one could be used with the others. The clothes were all of good quality, cleaned well and always looked like new garments. This young woman was meticulous in wearing fresh blouses, one of which served for informal dinner and evening wear.

Food. Food is frequently an item of unpredictable expense unless you are a careful watchdog of the treasury. In spite of fluctuating prices, hospitals in this country serve food that is usually adequate and well-balanced. You can save yourself much money as well as emotional wear and tear if you eat what is served and when it is served without "crabbing." You are fortunate if you are among the many young women of today who have been brought up to eat and like most foods and to eat regularly at meal times. If you have not been so fortunate, it might be worth your while to re-form your habits, since eating is much like any other routine habit and can, therefore, be moulded in large measure to a desired pattern through practice.

Recreation. Recreation is more important than some of us realize. "All work and no play makes Jack a dull boy," or, for that matter, Jill a dull girl. If you are to maintain good mental hygiene, recreation is essential, and good mental hygiene is basic to moral and physical well-being as well as to the prevention of personality quirks and instability. What form your recreation takes will depend both upon the school and upon yourself. Every school provides some type of extra-professional program. If your school program is restricted to one or two functions you will obviously need more outside diversion than if it is so comprehensive as to include most of the activities open to the young woman on the modern college campus. Then, too; your own likes and dislikes will affect the choice of forms of relaxation. One person may find relaxation in reading, another in sewing, in music or in sports. The important thing is to find out what, for you, affords the finest type of recreation and then to fit it into your budget. We recall one student in a medium-sized city who had little money for outside entertainment. She scanned the various papers, bulletins, and announcements and found that she could spend every hour of every day during the entire week in some form of free recreation, if she only had the time to spare. Not every situation will afford quite so varied a program, but planning and careful selection will usually yield inexpensive means of recreation for you. Perhaps in this field, as in that of eating, new desirable habits can be developed.

Professional Responsibilities

You are expected to be professional from the first day in school and from the first minute "on duty" this term "professional" will be set up before you as an ideal toward which to aim. What are some of its initial implications for you as a student?

Responsibility for Others. Possibly for the first time in your life you are now in a position in which you assume actual and growing responsibility for the care of others with all the ramifications that such responsibility entails. You assume obligation for helping to maintain health, to prevent illness, to relieve and cure disease. The saving of life itself is often in your hands. Patients rely upon you for the nursing service rendered them, as do their families and the physicians. As Dr. Edward L. Trudeau says, your aim is "to cure sometimes, to relieve often, to comfort always."

Here we might pause to indicate the qualities you require to assume such responsibility. Among the essential characteristics are integrity of character, broad tolerance, kindness, and a high sense of duty. Your aim should be to develop an integrity absolutely dependable in relation to patient care and to the recording of that care, which should always be as exact as a human can make them. No reason should ever be accepted as valid for incorrect care or for the inaccurate recording of it.

As important as integrity of character itself is a sense of broad tolerance. This may be evidenced through genuine respect for the personality, interests, and points of view of others, together with consideration for religions and races differing from your own. Kindness, entailing as it does a real liking for all manner of people—the rich and the poor, the halt, the lame and the blind—we may assume to be a prime quality of every nurse. Such kindness, however, should not be construed as mere sentimentality, but rather as a real understanding of the patient's needs and an adequate meeting of these needs without artificial dramatization.

We shall not attempt here to give a detailed description of all the personality traits which are valuable for good nursing, but simply stress the goal toward which all nurses work. The goal is that of good patient care in whatever situation the patient may be. The best way to develop the character of a good nurse is to assume the responsibility of giving, in as perfect a manner as possible, nursing care, or that segment of it for which you are prepared and to which you may be assigned. We believe that setting such a goal and working toward it to the best of your ability cannot fail to develop the traits of which we have been speaking. You cannot give good patient care without integrity, tolerance, kindness, and a sense of duty. Nor can you, for example, care rightly for your patients without exercising fine observation. And you are sure to engender in them, in their families, and in their physicians a sense of trust and faith in you. If you do your job of nursing rightly, assuming of course that you have ability and aptitude for it, these desirable traits of character will develop as by-products of your work and will stay with you for life.

Objectivity. Part of being a professional individual has to do with the quality of objectivity. Heretofore you have probably had little direct contact with suffering. Its first impact upon you is tremendous, particularly in case of serious injury or illness. You may tend, therefore, to identify yourself too closely with the patient and to react emotionally to even minor manifestations of his illness. Such a reaction would be encouraged if it were of help to the patient. Actually, the opposite is true, since in the presence of uncontrolled expressions of sympathy the patient, too, tends to react more emotionally than would otherwise be the case, as a child will weep when it sees its parents in tears. Psychologists tell us that for every stimulus there is a certain response. Your function, even as a beginning student, is to provide the stimulus which will draw forth the best reaction on the part of the patient. By your poise and calm you can contribute in no small measure to the patient's own calmness and confidence so necessary for his rest and, indeed, for his recovery.

Menial Tasks. In the average home there are many so-called menial tasks. They are performed in different ways. The real difference lies in the way they are done. In some homes children begin to help with home duties early because there seems to be a dignity about them, associated perhaps with their mother. Much of the beauty that clings about the memories of home life is due to this atmosphere of grace which hovers around the ordinary tasks of living. Unless your ideas of nursing have come entirely from the movies, you must be aware of the many simple duties involved in patient care. You know, too, that in nursing, as in the home, you may dispense these services with dignity and grace, because they are associated with the care of the patient and contribute to his welfare.

Professional Appearance. You will hear a great deal of stress put on professional appearance. Any uniform sets one apart. We like to think that the nurse's uniform is a source not only of comfort and practical convenience but also a source of protection to her and to the patient. The nurse going on a mission into a home at any hour of night and in the worst part of a large city is safe in her uniform. The public recognizes the uniform, knows something of what it symbolizes, and respects both it and its wearer.

Your complete indoor student outfit includes cap, uniform, apron (usually, though not always), shoes (with hose to match), and watch. Some schools will add pen, pencil and bandage scissors to this list. The cap, earned by students in most schools after a brief period in the school, is usually distinctive for the individual school as are also the uniform and the apron. Feet should be examined and proper shoes recommended by an orthopedic surgeon. Usually plain black or white shoes with medium heels are worn. The watch should have a second hand. The individual school usually indicates the type of watch preferred. In more recent years an attempt has been made to make the uniform attractive and comfortable while it remains plain and simple.

You will find that the greatest emphasis is placed upon being neat and trim at all times. Cleanliness of person and of clothing will rank at the top of the list of musts. Frequent shampoos, daily baths, neat hair, fresh cap, clean uniform (including collar, cuffs, apron, shoes, and stockings)—all these are quite as much in order as well cared for hands, good posture, and a well-modulated voice. The constant stressing of so commonplace a matter as cleanliness may at first be irksome to the student nurse and affect her much as it does a school boy. You may remember the story of how a foreign-born father came to a school, gave the name of his son, and asked to see him. The teacher said no child by that name was enrolled in the school. Persisted the father, "My Yohnny, he come by de school every day." Finally, the teacher suggested that he might recognize the child if he came up to the school room. This he did and pointed out his son. "No," said the teacher, "that is not your son. That is Johnny Govash." "Oh," said the father, "his mamma, she say 'Yohnny, go vash' in de morning, an' 'Yohnny, go vash' at noon, an' 'Yohnny, go vash' at night, till he tink his name is Yohnny Govash." You may feel for a while that at least your middle name must be Govash but you will get used to this and scrupulous scrubbing will soon become second nature with you.

Not only will you be told what to wear but also what not to wear. And among the "not to wear" will be found undue amounts of makeup, highly colored nail polish, jewelry of any kind (other than wedding ring and uniform watch), fancy hair dress, and in general anything that would tend to make you appear conspicuous. In addition, each school has regulations as to where or when the uniform may or may not be worn.

Some Suggestions. A number of other matters need only be mentioned, since a word to the wise nurse is sufficient. One who has had experience would probably suggest the following to the novice in the art of nursing:

1. Obey the doctor's orders, also the house rules. There are reasons. You will learn why later, if the reason is not immediately apparent.

2. Maintain quiet wherever patients are. Florence Nightingale said, "Unnecessary noise . . . is the most cruel absence of care."

3. Be professional with all patients.

4. Use discretion in your conversation with patients. Entertain and teach but remember that silence is somtimes golden.

5. Report even the slightest illness of your own at once. An ounce of prevention is worth a pound of cure. Incidentally you will avoid passing your infection on to others.

6. Keep your hands away from your face and wash them before meals. This procedure may prevent some of those "off-duty" days.

7. If you smoke, be careful not to do so in uniform. Stale tobacco smoke is obnoxious to most patients, even to those who themselves are smokers.

8. If you are dieting, do so only under the direction of a physician.

9. Refrain from eating food while on duty.

10. Avoid wasting hospital supplies. They cost money.

11. Work and play within reasonable limits. St. Vincent de Paul in the seventeenth century said, "It is a trick of the devil by which he gets good souls to do more than they can and so makes them unfit to do anything at all."

12. Live within your income. Refrain from borrowing.

> "Neither a borrower nor a lender be,
> For a loan oft loses both itself and friend;
> And borrowing dulls the edge of husbandry."

13. Cultivate good table manners.

14. Enjoy the beautiful—in nature and in music, literature and art. "A thing of beauty is a joy forever."

15. Cultivate many friends. But first to have friends you must be one.

16. Refrain from gossip. You have two eyes and two ears and one tongue that you may see and hear twice as much as you speak. Besides, most of what you would gossip

about has been entrusted to you in confidence. It is
not yours to relate.
17. Develop criteria for self-imposed authority. Better to
rule yourself than to be ruled by others.

Mental Hygiene

No list of the do's of adjustment to a successful nursing
career can be complete without some maxims of mental hygiene.
Your mental make-up is as important as your physical. We say,
"Take care of your health," and we should also say, "Preserve
a healthy outlook on life." In other words, success is so often
in proportion to the emotional drive you bring to your work
that the importance of the emotions cannot be overestimated.
Mental hygiene teaches how to control the emotions; how to
harness one's emotional force and make it work for one; how to
prevent it from standing in one's way.

The student who learns to "forget it" instead of allowing a
hurt to nag at the evenness of her disposition is gaining in
power. So is the one who takes pains to be especially cheerful
on a dark day. It is of paramount importance to get hold of bad
states of mind early before we have opportunity to develop
habitually bad attitudes. If we find ourselves with any undesirable feelings, we should try to change them before they
become recurrent. For example, if a student finds herself deciding that everyone is against her, that the instructor never
gives her a break, and that she could make good grades if she
did a bit of "apple polishing," she should immediately change
her attitude. Possibly the desired change may result from
thoughtful consideration of the situation after a good night's
sleep, or it may follow a talk with a friend or a trusted faculty
member. In extreme cases, she may feel the need of a mental
hygienist or even of a psychiatrist.

Another angle of the matter is that, concerning itself as it
does with the emotional life, mental hygiene differs for each
individual. Ironclad rules are, therefore, not universally applicable. All of us may learn from others, but each has a behavior pattern intrinsically her own, a pattern which can be
developed so as to include desirable attitudes and responses.

The nursing school period is, for most students, a time when many new attitudes and behavior patterns are being formed. The new environment with its complex situations presents to the young student many problems. These will not prove too much to cope with if the student approaches her problems in a constructive manner and forms the habit of thinking through her problems with a fair degree of objectivity.

Study Questions

1. Explain what is meant by "adjustment is a two-way process."

2. List some rules for intelligent adjustment.

Questions for Thought and Discussion

1. Make a budget of your time for one week. Try to live according to this plan.

2. At the end of a week's trial, review your time budget. Did you allow adequate time for study properly spaced? for other essential activities? If not, revise plan, seeking help of instructor or counselor, if desired.

3. Try setting up a budget of your money for a year, including an item for savings. Then try to live within the budget.

4. Outline your recreational program for the coming month. In what school activities do you plan to participate this year?

5. Discuss the statement, "Adjustment is a continuous process which goes on from birth to death."

6. Make a list of some good mental hygiene practices which you have found worked well.

7. How would you go about initiating a desirable change in residence regulations in your school?

Books to Read

A Curriculum Guide for Schools of Nursing. Section on Professional Adjustments, National League of Nursing Education, 1937.

Anderson, Camilla M.: *Emotional Hygiene* (*The Art of Understanding*). 3rd Ed. Philadelphia. J. B. Lippincott. 1943.

Beers, Clifford Whittingham: *A Mind That Found Itself: An Autobiography.* 25th Anniversary Edition. New York. Doubleday, Doran. National Committee for Mental Hygiene, 1935.

Cabot, Richard Clarke and Dicks, R. L.: *Art of Ministering to the Sick*. New York. Macmillan. 1936.

Clarke, Eric Kent: *Mental Hygiene for Community Nursing*. Minneapolis. University of Minnesota Press. 1942.

Diehl, Harold Sheely: *Healthful Living*. New Ed. Rev. New York. McGraw-Hill. 1941.

English, O. Spurgeon, and Pearson, Gerald H. J.: *Emotional Problems of Living: Avoiding the Neurotic Pattern*. New York. W. W. Norton and Co. 1945.

Krauch, Elsa: *A Mind Restored*. New York. Putnam. 1937.

IV

Intelligence in Nursing

INTELLIGENCE in nursing, as discussed here, is gauged by the manner in which you perform your regular or usual nursing duties. As a point of departure, let us survey the field of nursing activities with the aim of finding if there is not some well-marked line of differentiation between the ways in which they are done by various persons. It seems that such a study will reveal a line of demarcation, fluctuating but nonetheless existent, between two types of nursing. These types we would like to label as the "nurse-*in*-the-situation" and the "nurse-*to*-the-situation." In this we mark off a limited from a far-reaching, a shallow from a deep conception of the function of nursing. We mark off the nurse who is the technician from the real nurse. The real nurse is the one who exhibits intelligence in nursing.

Two Types of Nursing. The type of nursing done by the nurse technician, or nurse-*in*-the-situation, as we shall designate her, is familiar to all of us. Its content is primarily technique, and its aim is perfection of that technique. It is concerned only with carrying out specific and definitely ordered procedures in terms of technique. An illustration of this type of nursing may be seen in the work of a nurse who regards ward order as the *sine qua non* of effective service. She places primary emphasis upon such matters as neat appearance of the bed and uniformity in arrangement of room facilities. In such a routine matter as giving a patient a bath, this nurse's concern will be primarily to carry out the procedure and to do it as effectively and as quickly as possible.

The other type of nursing, that of the nurse-*to*-the-situation, has a more inclusive pattern. While it also includes the technical phases of nursing, it does not make of them an exclusive goal. It begins with technique but does not end there. This second type of nurse will likewise strive for order in the patient's room, but her concern will extend beyond this external phase to the total situation. If for any reason, a neat appearing bed makes for patient discomfort this nurse will be alert to the fact and correct it even though such action may result in ward disorder. A patient's comfort is more important than tightly tucked in covers. If the lowering of one of the window shades will lessen the light for a patient particularly sensitive to bright light, the shade will be drawn. In giving a bath, this second nurse will also aim at effective and rapid achievement. A good bath given rapidly may avoid unnecessary fatigue for the patient. But our second nurse's chief concern will not be with the bath alone, but with the patient's total pattern.

An illustration in this connection pertains to a private patient who upon entering the hospital a few days previously had been diagnosed as having typhoid. The patient, while being bathed one day, had become confidential with the nurse attending her and related to her a series of experiences having to do with an attempted abortion. The nurse was sufficiently alive to the significance of the patient's story to ask her to repeat this to the attending physician. This new information, confided at first to the nurse, led to a change in the diagnosis and, incidentally, to saving the patient's life, as the physician stated later. The nurse on the case was fortunately of the second type, i.e., a nurse-*to*-the-entire-situation, and exhibited intelligence in her nursing.

A further study of the differences between these types of nurses may paradoxically begin with a consideration of some ways in which they resemble each other. Take, for instance, the sources of their preparation. It is understood that both types of nurses draw their knowledge, skills, and perhaps even the attitudes which they apply in the nursing care of patients, from the same storehouses. Both types receive the same instruction in the biological, medical, and social sciences as well as in the science and art of nursing itself. Both study such subjects as anatomy, bacteriology, pharmacology, psychology, sociology, nutrition, and nursing. Perhaps both of them receive experience in such services as medical, surgical, obstetric, pediatric, psychiatric, and tuberculosis nursing. In other words, school of nurs-

ing facilities and resources have been at the disposal of both
alike. Yet at the conclusion of their program one student becomes a nurse-*in*-the-situation, and the other a nurse-*to*-the-
situation. The difference between them lies in the fact that in
the performance of their duties they draw in varying degrees
from the available sources of instruction and manifest varying
degrees of interest and concern for the total situation.

In making this comparison it must not be thought that we
underrate in any way the delimited work of the nurse technician. There may even be cases where her type of excellence
is actually required, in which her type of service would surpass
that of the other nurse. Nor would we deprecate the importance
of careful detailed work. Our aim is merely to point out that
there is a danger of letting this emphasis on technique become
an end in itself and of excluding the greater values which should
inhere in the nursing service.

*The Nurse-*TO-*the-Situation*. During the rest of this discussion,
our interest will center upon the nurse who has the broader view
of her duties rather than upon the one who is merely a technician, important though the latter may also be. Let us see the
kind of nursing care which our nurse of the broader outlook may
be expected to give. There are six essential areas from which
the nurse-*to*-the-situation derives her effectiveness: character,
extra-professional activities, the biological sciences, the medical
sciences, the social sciences, and the nursing and allied arts.
Just what has this nurse, as she ministers at the bedside of a
patient, acquired in her preparation from these sources?

First, the resources found within the nurse herself, her habits
of living and thinking. As we have said, what the nurse brings
to the art of nursing will determine in large measure her contribution to the patient's care. Closely allied to the nurse herself
are those accomplishments which she gained from her extra-
professional program, where she has learned many definite
skills. In the extra-professional program she develops new
interests and desirable traits. Through such sports as swimming,
she has acquired grace and poise. Through a knowledge of
music or appreciation of art shared with patients, she helps
wonderfully to transform ill days into happy days. Her extra-
professional program, involving many group activities, has

Social Sciences
History of Nursing
Professional Adjustments
Psychology
Sociology
Economics
Political Science

Nursing and Allied Arts
Medical & Surgical Nursing (including communicable and venereal disease and tuberculosis)
Nursing Including Personal Health
Nursing of Children
Obstetric Nursing
Psychiatric Nursing
Public Health

Nurse

Extra-Professional Activities

Biological Sciences
Anatomy
Chemistry
Microbiology
Physiology

Medical Sciences
Introduction to Medical Science
Pharmacology

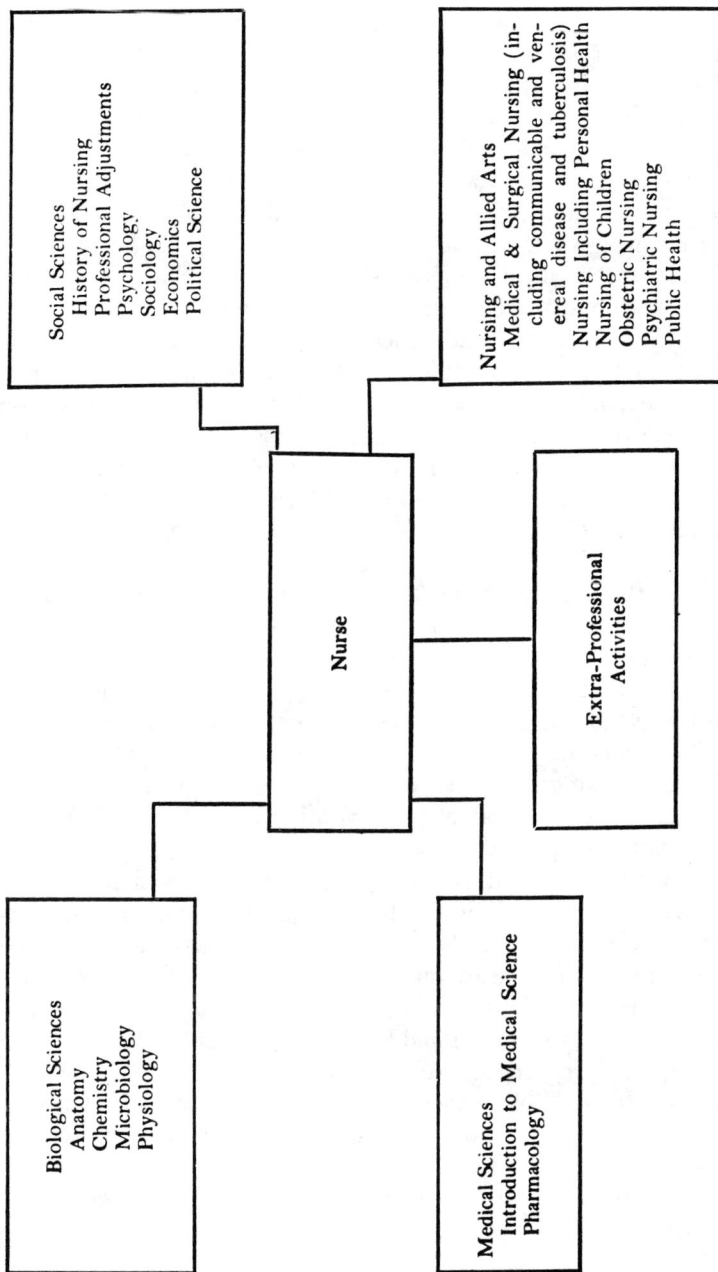

THE MAKING OF A NURSE

broadened her appreciation of community life. It has also deepened her sense of social and civic responsibility.

From the biological sciences she has learned the structure and functions of the body, and has come to understand something of the chemistry of digestion, together with the function of carbohydrates, fats, and proteins in bodily economy. She also has acquired information about pathogenic bacteria, and methods of preventing their spread.

From the medical sciences she has come to appreciate the significance of disease as an individual, community, and national problem. She understands such matters as the importance of vital statistics, the scientific methods used in modern medicine, and has been impressed with the need for accuracy of observation and recording. From this field also she has learned at first hand something about drugs, their sources, and their therapeutic actions and toxic effects upon the different systems of the body. She also appreciates the social significance of the indiscriminate use of drugs.

From the social sciences she has learned the implications for health of such a factor as low income. She has acquired an appreciation of the need to understand psychological processes and to practice good mental hygiene. She has also developed sensitivity to the opportunities and responsibilities of a professional person.

From nursing and the allied arts, she has developed an appreciation of the value of preventive as well as of curative work, both as applied to the individual and to groups. She has learned and practiced actual nursing in various fields taking cognizance the while of both the physical and mental concomitants of this care. She has acquired a knowledge of the important part played by nutrition in the welfare of her patient. Her experience has ranged from attending patients needing such simple nursing as feeding and bathing to those receiving oxygen therapy or intravenous treatments.

Illustrations. While cases without number occur illustrating the way in which the nurse adaptable to the situation is keen to draw upon what she has garnered from all these six sources, it may be sufficient here to indicate briefly how she applies this knowledge.

A patient is convalescing from an illness. The nurse may meet spontaneously certain almost unfelt needs of the patient, if she has resources within herself such as come from fine living and thinking. An example of this is the case of a nurse who cared for an elderly patient through a long period of convalescence. At no time was the subject of religion discussed, yet the patient stated one day that although he had never been a churchgoing man, he would like to become a member of the church to which the nurse belonged.

Again, a child patient needs diversional therapy. In this case, the nurse will not be satisfied with a mere routine of varied activities. She will bring into play much of what she has learned in developing her own leisure time skills and will offer intelligent guidance of the patient in developing new interests and attitudes.

To a child patient with a preventable communicable disease the nurse gives not only the required care that has been ordered, but she may go even beyond this. She knows something of the nature of the bacteria involved and of prevention of their spread. She inquires about the other children in the family. She may talk over with the mother the desirability of their immunization, and advise her of the service of community health agencies. She is not satisfied until she knows that, in addition to the patient being cared for in the hospital, the family and community are being protected also.

Suppose we have a patient suffering severe pain. Both the doctor and the nurse know the patient must have the required sedatives. Both know also something of the implications of too long use of such drugs. Further, both know that good nursing may often be a substitute for medication. The nurse who can make the patient comfortable both physically and mentally has carried the patient far toward his recovery without unnecessary medication.

Again, the patient is suffering from a deficiency disease. The nurse will be concerned not only with giving the patient the required physical care in the hospital, but she will also be sensitive to the many factors within the patient's life and in the community which produced the condition. She will do whatever she can to correct the situation and so exert her influence in favor of prevention as well as of cure.

Lastly, suppose a patient comes into the hospital for an operation. Feeling inadequate in a new and strange environment and unhappily anticipating the atmosphere of an operating room, the patient is restless, unstrung, apprehensive. The doctor leaves orders concerning the patient's diet, medication, and treatment. The nurse-*to*-the-situation carries out these orders, but in so doing she also manages to reassure the patient. She interprets the doctor's orders in such a way as to instil into the patient unqualified confidence in the doctor. She explains enough of operating room routine to allay unnecessary fear of tomorrow's experience. She transfers to her charge a sense of the interest of all hospital personnel in his welfare and sends to the operating room a patient who is calm, trusting, and secure in the feeling that his welfare is in competent and interested hands. This removal of anxiety will contribute in no small measure to the success of the operation.

It is in the hospitals, in the homes, wherever she is called upon, that the nurse-*to*-the-situation responds to the total needs of the case. In countless ways intelligence touches and illumines her regular duties. The highest qualities of personality and character are tested in the various situations a nurse may face.

Study Questions

1. What is meant by "intelligence in, nursing"?
2. What is meant by "a nurse who is merely a technician"?
3. Explain your concept of a "nurse-*to*-the-situation."

Questions for Thought and Discussion

1. Give an example from your own experience in which your nursing care of a patient exceeded the assignment made to you by the head nurse, because you applied intelligence to the situation.

2. Give an example from your own experience of how you "nursed the patient's mind" while giving physical care to his body.

3. Give an example of how you used an opportunity to teach a significant health concept or attitude to a patient, even though you had not planned to teach this particular thing.

4. Give an example of how symptoms which you observed in

a patient in the hospital probably arose from conditions existing at home.

5. Give an example of how symptoms which you observed in a patient in the hospital probably were aggravated by conditions existing at home, such as lack of food, unsatisfactory family relationships.

Books to Read

American Council on Education: Nursing Education for National Service. The Council. 1942.

Goodrich, Annie Warburton: *Social and Ethical Significance of Nursing: A Series of Addresses*. New York. Macmillan. 1932.

Nutting, Mary Adelaide: *Sound Economic Basis for Schools of Nursing, and Other Addresses*. New York. Putnam. 1926.

V

Legal Responsibilities

Pᴇʀʜᴀᴘs ʏᴏᴜ recall the sensation when, for the first time, you
looked at an x-ray picture of the human body. It scarcely seemed
possible that you had looked at persons all your life without
ever being aware of their inner framework. Similarly, the ordinary business of living runs along so uneventfully that one
seldom contemplates the solid legal framework which supports
and protects the person in every ramification of his social existence. Your security depends upon laws which afford fire and
police protection; laws that control the water and milk supply,
as well as sanitation in general, to mention only a few matters
pertaining to your existence in a complex society. Yet one
seldom thinks of these legal safeguards and is perhaps even
unaware of them.

So it is in the narrower sphere of your activity as a nurse.
When you enter the profession, you, as an individual, accept
wholeheartedly the *moral* responsibility of doing everything
possible for the patient's welfare and probably give little
thought to the legal implications of the nurse-patient relationship. But you also bear *legal* responsbility in case you should do
something which might bring harm to the patient. No one
should knowingly harm another person, if all are to be secure
in life and the pursuit of happiness, but the nurse is not permitted
to do so *even unknowingly*.

As a student you are responsible for your nursing acts, though
probably you would never be held liable in a court of law except
in cases of gross negligence (which might be of the nature of
either omission or commission), or in criminal cases, such as
sanctioning or assisting in an illegal abortion, for which you
are at all times responsible.

Where, then, does the chief legal responsibility for the

patient rest? Perhaps you assume that this belongs to the hospital, to the public health agency, or to the individual doctor. This is often the case. The private hospital, for instance, is held legally responsible for all acts (other than those of a criminal nature) committed by both student and graduate nurses. A charitable institution, however, can be sued only if it can be proved that it has not exercised due care in the selection of its personnel.

The Student Nurse's Legal Responsibilities

But what is your own responsibility in the institution in which you are studying nursing? When, as a student, you accept the privilege of learning nursing, do you not at the same time also accept the implied responsibility of practicing it with the greatest regard for safety? You have undoubtedly seen a pharmacist dispensing drugs. You have observed how cautiously he balances the amount of the drug on one pan against the exact required weight on the other. Just so nicely must your sense of personal responsibility match your privilege. Let us, therefore, not waste time over the significance of the legal term *responsibility*, but let us be clear in our minds that, though the hospital, public health agency, or the doctor bear the full brunt of this responsibility, you as a student should act as if you had an equal share in it, as you actually will have later when you work independently as a graduate nurse.

The question naturally presents itself: For what can the institution where you are studying nursing be held legally responsible? In general, it would be responsible for anything which brings harm to the patient. To particularize, we may list a few of the more common dangers of possible harm to the patient. By being aware of them and exercising special care you will contribute greatly to the protection of both your patient and the hospital.

Doctor's Orders. To begin with, there is the well known and important matter of doctor's orders. These should be written out in advance so as to avoid any possible misunderstanding or error. It is well for you to remember that the administration of a wrong medication or the omission of an important one may form the basis for a lawsuit against the hospital. You can pre-

vent such legal action by carrying out a doctor's order meticu-
lously, or, when wrong medication has been ordered as,
fortunately, happens very rarely, by calling the doctor's attention to this fact. It is well for you to remember that you as well
as the physician could be held legally responsible in any situation
arising from the administration of a harmful drug.

Much more rarely a situation may develop in which you feel
that your patient is not receiving proper or adequate medical
treatment. In such an event, usually the best thing to do is to
report your apprehension to the head nurse, or to the instructor,
who in turn may gain the necessary cooperation to secure
proper care either directly through the physician in charge, or
through consultation.

Burns. Next, we must consider the matter of causing burns.
Burns may be caused by such means as hot compresses, hot
water bottles, hot solutions, or by thermoelectric treatment
(electric light bulbs, and so on). These are so easily preventable
that it is practically inexcusable negligence to cause them. All
that one ordinarily needs to do is to exercise *due care* in the use
of materials and to observe carefully their effect upon the patient. In the case of hot compresses, for example, be sure they
are perfectly dry. In the use of hot water bottles, or hot solutions, safety will in most cases be assured by adjusting the heat
to the desired temperature with the aid of a thermometer. In
thermoelectric treatments it is essential to follow carefully the
doctor's orders as to amount and length of treatment, and then
to observe carefully and report the patient's reaction to it. In
rare instances, patients are unable to tolerate even the slightest
heat. On the other hand, they may be insensitive to the highest
temperature. These unusual cases require most careful observation and reporting.

Narcotics. The matter of handling narcotics is of such paramount importance in medical and nursing practice that it is
essential for the nurse to be very familiar with the Harrison
Narcotic Act designed as a protection for everyone concerned.
The purpose of the act is to regulate the "manufacture, sale,
dispensing, and prescribing of narcotic drugs."* Its most im-

* Wright, Harold, and Montag, Mildred, *A Textbook of Materia Medica,
Pharmacology, and Therapeutics*, 3rd Ed., pp. 154–156.

portant provisions will be found in your pharmacology text-book.

The nurse, student or graduate, has little if any responsibility so far as the purchase, dispensing, and prescribing of narcotics is concerned, since the hospital, agency, or doctor handles these matters under the terms of the law. *It is even illegal for her to have narcotics in her possession at any time,* except as she acts directly under a doctor's orders. She is, of course, responsible at all times for administering narcotics under the doctor's orders and must *herself* record all such medication on the patient's chart. She is also expected to conform to the system set up for the care of narcotics in the place in which she is working. It is her duty to report immediately to her superior officer any irregularity in the purchasing, dispensing, prescribing, or recording of habit-forming drugs. The following story is pertinent as an illustration of proper behavior in a situation involving the illicit use of narcotics. In a certain hospital a nurse student noted that her name had been signed on a chart for the administration of morphine. Actually, she had not given the drug. She checked back and found several similar entries on charts signed with her name. She learned that a graduate nurse on the station had been taking the tablets, recording these on the charts of the patients on the floor under the signature of the student nurse. The student reported the matter at once to the director of the school with the result that the pernicious practice was stopped at once. The guilty nurse was placed immediately under medical care and was later able to return to responsible nursing work. Had not her habit of taking drugs been detected early, and promptly reported, it is doubtful if she could have regained her usefulness as a nurse.

Charts. Probably one of the first things to be impressed upon a nurse student's mind is the importance of accurate and intelligent charting. Some hospitals file all nursing charts as part of the permanent record. More hospitals would probably follow such a practice if the nurse's charting could be made more intrinsically valuable. A few hospitals discard all nurses' charts. We wish to point out here that the nurse's record of a patient's care and treatment is often used in court in cases of alleged malpractice, and may therefore contribute important evidence

in deciding a legal contest. A few examples may be cited as
illustrations. A patient brought suit against a hospital for neglect of care. Among other things he stated that he had had no
bath during his stay in the hospital and that he had had no
medical examination preceding an operation. By way of explanation, it may be said that the patient interpreted a bath as
being a tub bath and a medical examination as being one given
him on the ward. Through some error, a record of the doctor's
examination was not attached to the chart. The nurse's chart,
however, showed that nursing care including bed baths had been
given as ordered and that the physician's examination had been
completed in the outpatient department just previous to the
patient's admission to the hospital proper. This case was won
by the hospital largely because there was a record in the nurse's
chart of the actual care received by the patient. Another point
is the need of recording on a patient's chart immediately upon
admission the presence of pressure sores. If this is done, the
hospital may be spared much worry and even troublesome
litigation.

Patient's Effects. Much time and anxiety, too, may be spared
for everyone if all clothing and valuables are fully listed, as the
following incident will show. A critically ill patient was once
admitted to the hospital. The patient was wearing a valuable
diamond ring. In the hurried effort to get the patient cared for
promptly no mention was made of the ring on the admission
chart. When the patient was ready to leave the hospital the ring
was missing. The nurse was sure that the family had taken the
ring. The family, on the other hand, was equally positive that
the ring was lost in the hospital and insisted it would bring
suit unless the ring was returned or paid for. Only with great
difficulty and persistent effort, in view of the fact that the life
of the patient on admission hung in the balance and that concern
with such matters as a ring would have jeopardized the primary
object of saving the patient's life, was the family finally per-
suaded to drop the case. A moment's time and a bit more alertness on the part of the admitting nurse or student would have
averted the whole troublesome incident.

Although a student will practically never be implicated in a
lawsuit, the following incident illustrates how a student may

occasionally become involved in a legal situation. A patient turned over a sum of money to his brother in the presence of a student who was taking care of him. The student did not know whether this was a gift or was given for safe keeping. It so happened that the brother died shortly thereafter, and his family believed that the money had been given to him as a gift. The patient brought suit to recover the money from his deceased brother's family. Both parties to the litigation wished to call in the nurse as a witness for their side. She was advised to request "privileged communication," which, if granted, would mean that she could not be forced to divulge confidential information given her in line of duty. Had this privilege not been granted by the court and had she been summoned as a witness in the case, her duty would have been simply to state the bare facts truthfully and objectively but not interpret them in any way.

Accidents. Still another illustration will demonstrate the many legal complications which may arise from the administration of hospital care. One winter day a small child was struck down by an automobile in front of her home. Fortunately, a student from a nearby hospital happened to come by at the time. The student at once reported the accident to the director of her school, who notified the hospital and the police. The unconscious child was not moved though it lay in the street. It was covered warmly but left undisturbed until the hospital ambulance arrived on the scene. It was then cautiously lifted on splints and placed in the ambulance, together with its mother. The student remained at the scene of the accident until the injured child was turned over safely to medical hands. At the hospital the child was examined very carefully and all the observations were recorded in detail. The examination revealed that the child suffered a skull fracture and a spine injury. In caring for the child it was necessary, among other things, to shave her hair (for which the mother's permission was duly obtained) and its clothes were removed by having them ripped.

This incident includes several elements involving legal responsibility. First, the accident was immediately reported, which is fundamental and very essential. Time saved may mean a life saved. No matter how insignificant the accident it should be reported at once. Then, the injured child was given every possible attention, it was kept warm and unmoved even though it was lying on the street pavement in winter. Also, the nurse stayed with the child until medical aid arrived. In addition to the careful examination of the child's condition and recording the findings, the mother's permission was obtained to cut the child's hair. And, finally, the clothing was ripped, not cut. Any one of these items and many more, if handled differently or overlooked, could have furnished a basis for legal action and caused costly litigation.

Witnessing a Will. We should not conclude this chapter on legal responsibility without at least brief mention of the making of a will by a patient. Occasionally a nurse is asked to witness a will. The drawing of a will is governed by statute and definitely laid down rules. The nurse should be familiar with the three fundamental tests of the validity of a will. First, was the will properly executed? Second, was the person making the will of sound mind? Third, was the will written freely or under compulsion? A will must be attested by two persons to have legality. In the case of a patient, a lawyer ought to draw up the will if there is still enough time to make the proper arrangements. A statement of a patient on the death-bed will be admitted in court provided the patient was aware that he was dying. If the patient desires to make a will but his mind is no longer lucid, then both a doctor and a lawyer should be present at the drawing of the document.

An incident will illustrate the assistance a nurse may be called upon to give in connection with the making of a will. A patient who had been injured in an automobile accident late one evening was brought to the hospital for care. During the night he asked the nurse to write a note to his absent wife saying goodbye and stating that he wished all his property to go to her. Since the patient felt there was not time to wait for a doctor or a lawyer, the nurse made a verbatim record of the patient's request, which was accepted as a legal document. As such it facilitated the transfer to the wife of all the patient's property without loss of time or money.

The nurse by virtue of her activity and in line of regular duty, frequently stands in very intimate relation to the patient who is grievously ill or is on the brink of death. She may quite involuntarily and not at all by choice become a witness to the dying person's wishes or to the actions of relatives who survive him. The good nurse will know that she has a great moral responsibility in such matters, besides the purely legal one. If called upon, she should discharge that responsibility in the noblest tradition of her profession.

Study Questions

1. What do you think is the difference between moral responsibility and legal responsibility for the patient's welfare? Which do you consider to be the greater responsibility?
2. What is the legal responsibility of a private, as contrasted with a charitable institution?
3. Explain the three fundamental tests of the validity of a will.
4. What is meant by "privileged communication"?

Questions for Thought and Discussion

1. Assemble for study as many as possible of the rules and regulations of the hospital in which you are having clinical experience. Do you think that some of these rules of procedure are intended to protect the patient from harm? Which regulations are intended to guard the hospital from unjustified legal suits?
2. Dr. Jones and Dr. Smith each have a patient with lobar pneumonia in the ward where you are on duty. Dr. Jones has ordered sulfadiazine for his patient; Dr. Smith has not ordered this medication for his patient. Dr. Jones' patient is getting well; Dr. Smith's patient is apparently not progressing well. Should you, as the nurse, conclude that Dr. Smith's patient is being neglected? If so, why? If not, why not?
3. There is a hospital regulation in the hospital where you are on duty which prohibits nurses from accepting verbal orders for medicines to be given to patients. One of your patients has suddenly taken a turn for the worse and you have telephoned to the doctor to report the change in condition and to receive instructions. The doctor has ordered by telephone an emergency medication. Would

you refuse to give this medication because of the hospital rule regarding verbal orders? If you refuse, have you discharged your responsibility to the patient? If you carry out the order, have you discharged your responsibility to the hospital? How is your responsibility to the patient and the hospital's responsibility to the patient the same? In what ways do these two responsibilities differ?

4. Can you cite instances in which a nurse's chart has been used in a law suit? What use was made of the chart? Of what value was the evidence provided by the nurse's record?

5. List some of the ways in which you as a student may help to prevent legal action being necessary against your hospital.

Books to Read

Hoyt, Emanuel, and Hoyt, L. R.: *Legal Guide for American Hospitals.* Hospital Textbook Company. 1940.

Oppenheimer, Benton S.: *Treatise on Medical Jurisprudence.* Baltimore. Wm. Wood. 1935.

Scheffel, Carl, and McGarvah, Eleanor: *Jurisprudence for Nurses,* 2d ed. Chicago. Lakeside Press. 1938.

VI

Student and Professional Organizations

In theory, at least, the democratic way of life presupposes a participation of every citizen in the various activities of the community. Of course, one could not possibly find the time, nor would one be temperamentally inclined to participate in every activity constituting the life of the community. All, however, have the responsibility for solving problems and for being alert to the preservation of their rights and interests, since the successful working of a democratic society presupposes that none shall take an attitude of indifference, sit aside and leave responsibility to the few. True, a few will bear major responsibility for the administration of government. These are the elected officers and representatives who are the instruments through which the citizens continue to express their will. But the important thing is that in a democracy authority ultimately must rest in the large body politic which merely delegates responsibility, without relinquishing it, to its elected representatives.

Thus to be good citizens under the democratic way of life, we must learn above all else to live with our neighbors. We cannot, as Daniel Boone did in an earlier day, move away every time anybody settles within twenty miles of us. We have to learn to govern ourselves and to accept graciously the decision of the majority. In the democratic way, we willingly accept sacrifices for the greater gifts which this brings. If on the one side of the scale is found responsibility, on the other side is liberty with all its blessings. Under normal conditions, at any rate, we as adults are very largely free to determine the way in which the nation, the state, the locality, or some of the smaller groups to which we belong may go.

Authority for group action lies within the group itself. To implement this authority the group selects its own representatives to draw up laws. The orderly existence of the group depends upon abiding by the rules laid down by the majority. Commensurate with the privilege of self-government is the responsibility which each of us has for its successful functioning. In a democracy you are not born to the privilege. You do not spring full-fledged and overnight into full citizenship. It is something that you must grow into.

Participation in a student government organization is one of the best means of promoting this growth. If, as an adult, you are to live effectively as a citizen in a democracy, it will help greatly if, as a student of nursing, you have served an apprenticeship in learning the art of democratic living.

Organizing Student Government. Let us, therefore, consider first the organization for student self-government. This organization is usually composed of all students in the school, although entering students oftentimes do not have full privileges (or responsibilities) until after some stated period of residence in the school. Since you may have already participated in a similar organization either in high school or college, you probably will be familiar with the general procedure of drafting a constitution and by-laws, as well as with drawing up house rules and regulations. In any event, some faculty member or your alumnae president will be glad to assist with the essential details of organization.

In your student organization, the constitution will probably contain a definite statement of its purpose; method of administration, including a list of elected officers and their prescribed duties; the franchise, indicating conditions of voting and election; the calling of meetings; and amendments. By-laws implement the basic principles and provisions of the constitution. They deal with finances (dues and budget), standing committees, and other phases of the organization which may be changed more frequently than the provisions contained in the constitution. House rules usually form a separate set of enactments and will vary greatly from school to school depending upon local conditions.

Even the purpose of the student organization may vary. Generally, it will have to do primarily with the so-called extra-professional part of the nursing program, but in many schools it may also cover curriculum problems. But regardless of these differences, which depend upon the individual school, basically every student organization will be concerned with fostering unity of spirit and purpose in the student body, promoting co-operation between students and faculty, and stimulating and directing social and cultural activities in the school.

In carrying out these objectives a student organization, in cooperation with the faculty, will strive to engage every student in the school in some type of social activity and, unless contra-indicated by health conditions, also in some field of sports. The organization will see to it that every entering student, if she so desires, shall have a "big sister" to guide her. It will also take care that such group activities as teas, picnics, and musicals occur at frequent intervals. But perhaps most important of all, through a publication or some other medium, it can make vocal student opinion or needs and thus furnish a very essential link in the mutual relationship between the students and the faculty. Conducted along democratic lines, and supported wholeheart-edly by the entire student body, such an organization may be instrumental in bringing about much needed improvements in the school.

A few words may also be said about the technique of putting into effect the purpose of the organization. The meetings of the organization are conducted in accordance with a set of rules known as parliamentary law, which is one of the greatest achievements of our modern civilization. Participation in a stu-dent organization in which there is an opportunity to practice parliamentary law affords excellent training in the qualities es-sential to the democratic way of life. Because of its important social implications, this technique will be discussed in some detail.

Parliamentary Law

Human beings (at least some of them) found after many cen-turies of bitter experience that in the long run they could ob-tain more happiness in life by letting their group action be determined by the will of the majority instead of by the irre-sponsible will of some leader who happened to possess power because of an impressive physique, an eye that none might brook, an engaging personality, inherited wealth, or social position—traits or circumstances which do not imply either brains or conscience. Men also found that the will of the majority is still more likely to be right if that majority is in a cool, rational state of mind when they are in the process of "willing." Parliamentary law is designed to secure this rational state, for rationality consists in judging a question by giving heed to all the arguments on both sides and excluding irrelevant personal and emotional considerations. Rules of order do more than provide the machinery for the majority to register their will: they promote intelligent judgments by securing a hearing for the minority, so that all possible views may be presented before a decision is reached. Thus parliamentary law is the keystone to democracy, tolerance, rationality, and progress. Through it intelligence prevails over blind, animal impulse and emotion.

In ordinary meetings only a few rules of procedure are needed. Yet it is important that these few be known by all students, not only for their own protection in meetings, but also for the promotion of democratic and rational group action in general. After mastering the rules given here, any students desiring a more complete knowledge of the subject may find it in Roberts' *Rules of Order*.

Conduct of a Meeting

Opening a Meeting. The chairman of an assembly opens a meeting by saying, "The meeting will please come to order." She then says, "The secretary will please read the minutes of the preceding meeting." After the secretary has finished reading, the chairman says, "Are there any corrections to the minutes?" If, after a slight pause, no member points out any inaccuracy in the minutes, the chairman continues, "If not, they stand approved as read." She then asks whether there is any old business or states what old business is to be taken up. Any committees appointed at a previous meeting to investigate some question now report, and any other matters left over from the preceding meeting are disposed of. The chairman then says, "We shall now proceed to the orders of the day," or "The meeting is now open to any new business which anyone cares to bring up."

If an organization has previously adopted a definite order of business, or if the officers or the executive committee have been authorized to prepare the agenda for each meeting, this order of business must be followed. After each item is completed, the chairman announces the next topic. *A question can be taken up out of its regular order only by a two-thirds vote.*

Obtaining the Floor. In order to obtain the floor, a member rises and says, "Madam Chairman." The chair recognizes the member, that is, allows her to speak, either by nodding to her, in small informal meetings, or by saying, "Miss——," mentioning the member's name. If members are not acquainted with each other, a member in obtaining the floor should state her name when the chairman pauses after "Miss."

If several members rise at the same time, the chairman should decide between them with fairness to both sides of the debate. It is best to alternate between the two sides in granting the floor. Also the same person should not be given the floor twice until every member has had a chance to speak. If the chairman does not know in advance the sides which members are likely to take and if it happens that all the persons recognized have spoken on the same side, she should say, "are there any views on the other side of this question which someone would like to present?"

The chairman is not entitled to debate a question but must act merely as a referee without giving any intimation of her own views. If she feels that she must air her opinions, then it is necessary for her to resign her chair, at least until the pending question is settled. In less formal meetings, however, it is permissible for the chairman to express her opinion after most of those desiring to speak have done so.

Making a Motion. After obtaining the floor and after giving some preliminary arguments, a member wishing to make a motion says, "I move that we do so-and-so." (It is better form to say, "I move," than to say "I make a motion.") The chairman then says "It is moved that we do so-and-so. Is there a second to the motion?" If anyone cares to second the motion, she simply says, "I second it." It is not necessary to rise and secure the floor in order to second a motion. The chair next says "It is moved and seconded that we do so-and-so. Is there any discussion?" The question is then open for debate. If a motion is not seconded, the chairman simply calls for other business.

After a motion has been seconded, it is before the house and cannot be withdrawn by the mover without the consent of the seconder, or without the permission of a majority of the members, in case it is so important that some member insists on its remaining before the house.

Amending a Main Motion. It is very important for both the chairman and the members to think clearly when an amendment of a main motion is attempted. The cardinal point to remember is that, when an amendment is proposed and seconded, the amendment must be debated and voted on first *by itself.* If the amendment is adopted, this simply means that the motion before the house is restated, and is ready for debate in its new form as amended. If the amendment is not adopted, this means that discussion on the motion as originally stated is to be resumed. Do not confuse voting on an amendment with voting on the whole question. The correct procedure is something like this: A member moves to amend a motion (by adding, deleting, or substituting certain words, phrases, or sentences). The motion is seconded and the chairman says, "It is moved and seconded that the motion be amended in such and such a way. Is there any discussion?" After some discussion, the chairman says, "All those in favor of the amendment, say 'Aye'; those opposed, 'No.' The ayes have it. Is there any further discussion on the motion as amended?" After the discussion has ended, the chairman finally puts the main question as amended to a vote.

Speeding up Action. Sometimes the debate on a question drags out to such an extent that the best interests of a meeting require that it be stopped. There are several legitimate methods of doing this. *One is to limit debate to so many minutes per speaker. This requires a two-thirds vote.* Another method is to move "the previous question." Moving the previous question is simply moving that a vote be taken on the main question without further debate. *When the previous question has been moved and seconded, it must be voted on at once without any debate. A two-thirds vote is required in order to carry this motion.* If the motion does carry, the chairman is thereby compelled to call for a vote on the main question at once without any further debate whatsoever.

In informal meetings it is usually not necessary to move the previous question, but when most of the members feel that the question has been debated sufficiently, someone says "Question!" and, if silence ensues, the chairman says, "If there is no further discussion, we will vote on the question." Sometimes, however, certain persons, who never seem to recognize a real need for debate, make a nuisance of themselves by always shouting "Question!" In such cases, the chairman should call them to order.

In some bodies, which conduct an enormous amount of business, as the House of Representatives, and have a definite division of members into majority and minority parties, time is saved by moving "to lay on the table" such motions as are sure to be defeated. *A motion to lay on the table is voted on at once, cannot be debated, and requires only a majority vote.* It is generally not fair to use such procedure in an ordinary meeting, and students should rarely, if ever, use it, but should give the minority in every case a chance to express their views and then vote on the main question in the regular way. Laying on the table, however, sometimes serves the useful purpose of saving an organization from going on record for or against a proposition, when it is the consensus of the meeting that such evasion is best for the time being. Laying on the table is also a useful device, especially when accompanied by a specific directive as to when the motion is to be taken up again, in cases where a more representative or informed vote can be obtained at a later date.

Voting. Voting may be done in ordinary cases by acclamation. That is, the chairman may say, "All those in favor of the motion say 'Aye,' . . . those opposed, 'No,' and, if it is clear that the motion is carried, she says, "The motion is carried." In some cases, however, when the question is important or the vote close, it is necessary to have a show of hands, a standing vote, or even a secret ballot. Any member, if he thinks a vote of acclamation did not express the opinion of the meeting accurately, may call for a "division." The chairman is then compelled to ask for a show of hands or to take a standing vote, or, if demanded, a written vote, so that an exact count may be made. The chairman is not entitled to a vote except in the case of a tie.

Nullifying an Action. If a motion has been passed at a meeting and it is desired to repeal the action at the same meeting, there are two ways open. *One is for a member who voted for the measure to move "to reconsider" the measure. This motion requires only a majority vote but cannot be made by a member who was on the losing side.* The other form of repeal is one that is open to members on the losing side. *This is the motion "to rescind" the action. It requires a two-thirds vote.*

At a subsequent meeting any previous enactments of the society may be repealed by a simple majority vote, unless there is some provision in the constitution or by-laws prohibiting it.

Points of Order. If any member thinks that the chairman is not conducting the meeting according to parliamentary law, she may stand and say, "Madam Chairman, I rise to a point of order." The chairman must interrupt the proceedings at once and recognize the objector by saying, "Please state your point." After the point has been stated, the chairman, if she accepts the criticism, says, "The chair stands corrected." If she does not agree with the member's point, she says, "The objection is overruled," and states the reason for her ruling. If the member is still unconvinced, she may appeal the decision of the chair. The chairman must then put the point of order to a vote by saying, "All those in favor of sustaining the chair say 'aye,'" and so on.

Nominations. Nominations, unlike motions, do not require a second. Students waste a great deal of breath in unnecessarily seconding nominations at school elections.

A motion to close nominations requires a two-thirds vote. A knowledge of this fact may be useful in combatting school politicians. It is an old trick among college students to "fix" an election by arranging in advance to have their candidate nominated first and then in rapid succession to nominate some obscure student, for whom no one will vote, and then to move that the nominations cease, second the motion, and carry it before any one realizes what has happened. The choice then being between their candidate and an obscure candidate, they are sure to win. The chairman should rule such a hasty motion out of order. If this is not done, a member should call for a division, that is, insist on an exact count of votes, reminding the chair, that a two-thirds vote is required to close nominations.

Tellers are appointed by the chairman to count the ballots when a written vote is taken. It is customary and fair to appoint tellers from both sides in case factions happen to exist in an organization.

Adjournment. A motion to adjourn takes precedence over all other motions, must be voted on at once after being seconded, and is not debatable. The extraordinary privilege, however, which this motion has, of interrupting the business of a meeting at any point, should not be abused. If the chairman sees that such a motion is made purely for purposes of obstruction, she may refuse to entertain it.

Ordinary meetings usually adjourn by common consent without any formal vote on adjournment.

Records. The *secretary* of an organization should keep an accurate record of the proceedings in the minutes of each meeting. Every motion, the name of the member moving it, and the vote on it should be recorded.

The *treasurer* should likewise keep an itemized account of receipts and expenditures and not depend upon her memory. For her own protection, she should keep all bills and receipts.

Professional Organizations

Upon graduating from school the nurse should look forward to membership in professional organizations. Nurses have found, as have others too, that in a complex society much more can be accomplished to achieve the ideals of the profession and recognition of its proper place in the scheme of things, by working together in a group, than can be attained by individual effort. We live in an age when things are accomplished by banding together.

We may illustrate this fact in a lighter vein by relating the following story. You may have heard of the gentleman who flicked off flowers with his walking stick as he walked down a garden path. Finally he came upon a patch in which there were some bumblebees. He passed on without molesting the flowers in that spot. When he was asked why he left these flowers undisturbed, the gentleman's reply was, "Oh, they've an organization there."

It is a matter of great practical importance that nurses should actively support their own professional organizations. The aims, functions, activities, programs, and policies of these various organizations are designed to promote social welfare as well as the interests of the nurse herself. Among the organizations are the alumnae association, the American Nurses Association (ANA), the National League of Nursing Education (NLNE), and the National Organization for Public Health Nursing (NOPHN), the last three forming official national nursing organizations. The alumnae association forms your permanent tie with your Alma Mater. It may also, and usually does, serve as a stepping stone to participation in local, state, and national organizations. The ANA is the principal official professional organization, open to all graduate registered nurses. Its chief purposes have to do with the promotion of the professional and educational advancement of nurses in every proper way, with the dissemination of information about nursing, and with the bringing of nurses and nursing associations into communication with each other. The NLNE membership is made up of those engaged and of those interested in educational work in the field of nursing. It specializes in maintaining standards of nursing education for the preparation of both the undergraduate student of nursing and the graduate nurse student. The organization serves in an advisory capacity to all accredited schools in the country in such matters as curriculum, personnel, and administration.

The NOPHN is composed of lay persons, agencies, and nurses. The organization serves in an advisory capacity to the public health agencies and persons engaged in public health teaching and service with the view of upholding certain standards and developing newer practices in their field of activity.

We should also include here The International Council of Nurses (ICN), to which any member of the ANA automatically belongs. The ICN is concerned with promoting the welfare of the nursing profession the world over, serving as a clearing house for the exchange of ideas and fostering international friendship. Its meetings take place every four years in different countries.

Finally, we should mention The American Red Cross Nursing Service which acts as a reservoir of nurses who are willing to serve in times of emergency or disaster. This organization is one to which you will wish to belong when, as a graduate nurse, you are eligible for membership.

Study Questions

1. In what ways is active membership in a student organization preparing you for membership in your graduate professional organizations? Name the chief graduate professional organizations.
2. It is suggested that your class conduct meetings according to the outlined parliamentary procedure.
3. What are the advantages of parliamentary law?

Questions for Thought and Discussion

1. What are the purposes of your student organization?
2. "Authority for group action lies within the group itself." If a group of persons constitutes itself to take action in any situation, who should assume responsibility for the results of the group action?
3. What responsibility does your student organization place upon its members?
4. Enumerate activities carried on by your student organization and show how they contribute to desirable student growth and development.
5. Outline a plan whereby you as an individual may assist to the fullest in the development of democratic living within your group.
6. What means would you suggest for the further development of the democratic way of life within your own school?

Books to Read

Gannon, Ada K.: *Thumb Prints of Parliamentary Points.* The Author. 518 Victoria Building, St. Louis, Mo. 1934.

Harrison, Gene: *Professional Adjustments II.* St. Louis. Mosby. 1942.

Roberts, Henry Martyn: *Roberts' Rules of Order.* Scott Forsman and Co. 1915.

Spalding, Eugenia Kennedy: *Professional Adjustments in Nursing for Senior Students and Graduates.* 3d ed. Philadelphia. Lippincott. 1944.

PART II. PERSONAL, PROFESSIONAL, AND SOCIAL ETHICS

VII

Thinking About Ethics

It is a bitter pill for teachers of ethics to swallow but it is none the less true that most students, including students of nursing, approach a course in ethics with the expectation of being thoroughly bored. Nobody likes to be preached at— except maybe on Sunday when he is used to it. And nurses especially are likely to fall asleep over a book which tells them to practice the virtues of kindliness, patience, truthfulness, and so on, when it is perfectly obvious that they would not have been attracted into the nursing profession in the first place if they had not possessed those virtues in a high degree. Besides, anyone who is familiar with the curriculum of a school of nursing knows that in the course of her routine training a nurse will acquire numerous virtues, if she does not have them already, without needing to learn them out of a textbook in ethics. So students are right in expecting boredom from the study of ethics if it consists of nothing more than a preachment of the obvious.

There is another reason, too, why human beings in general— at least those in our own modern culture—shy away from sermonizing about ethics. We dislike self-righteousness and are suspicious of people who talk too much about morals. We have a feeling that they may be hypocritical. Also, paradoxically enough, even quite moral persons do not like to have the reputation of being *too* good. No student or teacher, for example, would consider it a compliment if he or she were introduced to a class as a very moral person. Any of us might like to be known as a good fellow, a nice girl, or a fine person but we would shrink from being called moral. Now this is partly due to a commendable modesty and partly due to the fact that many human beings are reared on traditional systems of morals which lay emphasis on the letter instead of the spirit of morality. In ethics we sometimes refer to outworn prohibitions found in these moral codes as *taboos*. They are often harmful and are not something which we develop within us in the sense that we may develop those qualities which a "nice girl" shows, etc. Young people have confused them with morality in the better sense of the word, and are skeptical for that reason about the entire subject of morals.

There is still another conception of ethics that has left many persons indifferent to the subject. Ethics is sometimes just a written code that some organization of business or professional people has worked out—to be framed, hung up on the wall, and promptly forgotten. Everyone knows that the code which is actually practiced is not to be found in books or engravings but in the general social atmosphere which surrounds any profession—a vague feeling communicated to apprentices so that they know what is expected of them. Memorizing rules that few, if any, feel under obligation to observe seems dull because it is unrealistic, a sanctimonious ritual having little relation to the world in which we live.

What Ethics Is. Yet ethics is not any of these things for which people have justifiably felt a distaste. It is not a preachment of pious platitudes, or of impossible virtues and uncritical taboos that most people "honor in the breach rather than in the observance," or of unrealistic, ornamental codes. Indeed, it is just because of our reactions against that mistaken sort of moralizing that we feel the need of another kind of ethics. If, for instance, we find that our traditional morality contains many prohibitions that very few people really respect, then it occurs to us that we need to discover some principle which we can use in revising our code—in separating the wheat from the chaff. How can we tell which of the rules that we have inherited from the past are harmful or at best useless? And how can we tell which rules represent sound human experience and wisdom? Again, if we find that professional codes are not workable or if there are border-line or emergency cases that are not dealt with by the written code, what principle are we to use in setting up a more realistic code or in using our discretion about making exceptions to a good general rule in certain exigencies? *Working out such a principle or standard by which we can judge both the original rules of conduct and the application of the rules is the proper business of an ethics course.* And the more one is dissatisfied with what is ordinarily called ethics, the more important it is for him or her to formulate an intelligent set of moral principles which will make ethics a vital and significant part of life.

The Nurse Who Thinks for Herself. But someone may say, "Yes, that is all right for people in general, but wouldn't it be rather dangerous for every nurse to work out her own rules of conduct for herself? Why should we expect every nurse to reach wise conclusions or the same conclusions? What would happen if every private in an army thought things out for himself? And is not the organization of a hospital necessarily somewhat similar to that of an army?" The answer to these questions is: yes and no. It is true that nurses are almost always a part of some organization. Many of their duties are determined for them in great measure by the hospital or other agency in which they work or by members of the medical profession with whom they work. No one would be so foolish as to advocate the anarchy of each nurse being a law unto herself. No organization, nor society in general, could function on that basis. But submitting to the necessary discipline of an organization does not prevent one from being intelligent about it, i.e., being able to think through the reasons for the rules which one observes, asking oneself whether they are wise or whether they just represent a tradition that no one has had the originality, energy, or courage to shake off. A free, rational person in a modern democratic society ought to be able to obey the rules of an organization and cooperate under them while at the same time passing private judgment upon them and resolving to improve them (when necessary) if given an opportunity.

Furthermore, new situations sometimes arise which no rule exactly fits, and if a nurse has thought through the general principles of ethics underlying all rules, she is more likely to be able to adopt a wise plan of action for the occasion. Seeing clearly what is at stake in choosing between two alternatives, she can make up her mind with confidence that she has done her best under the circumstances, having made full use of her intelligence in deciding what is the greater good or the lesser evil. Or, in the rare but very important cases that arise in which it would be stupid or fanatical to live up to the letter of the law, a nurse who has already done some reflecting on ethical problems will be able to make an exception with good reasons and an untroubled conscience. On the other hand, one who has never thought through any moral questions may sometimes impulsively do the right and the humane thing in breaking a rule but will be made unhappy by an unintelligent conscience which knows nothing but blind, undiscriminating obedience.

This does not mean, however, that a nurse or anyone else ought to go about constantly pondering the niceties and perplexities of ethical questions. This would only result in confusion and indecision, not to mention a great waste of time. Most of our decisions have to be made quickly on the basis of habits and rules of long standing. And any attempt to think through every bit of conduct, on the spot, would leave us in the same predicament as the self-conscious centipede:

> A centipede was happy quite
> Until a frog in fun
> Said, "Pray, which leg comes after which?"
> This raised her mind to such a pitch,
> She lay distracted in the ditch
> Considering how to run!

Thus, the time to do our critical ethical thinking is not when we are on the job but at other times when we can reflect at leisure and thresh out problems in conversation with ourselves, with our friends, with our teachers, or with the authors of books. The results of our reflection, then, can be held in reserve in the background of our minds, ready for some occasion which will require all the intelligence and originality that we have previously developed. Critical thinking carried on in this fashion does not reduce efficiency or undermine the discipline of an organization. Rather it increases efficiency by building up morale and self-respect.

There is another and last reason why nurses should be encouraged to do some philosophizing about moral principles. A nurse is not only a nurse. She is also a citizen and human being, and as such, particularly in a democratic society, she is entitled to speculate about anything under the sun in any way she pleases. No matter how rigid a discipline she may live under when on duty and no matter how little opportunity there may be to use her own discretion in some matters, there remain many hours when she exists as a private person who should be unhampered in her freedom of thought and even in her freedom of expression, provided that her manner of expressing herself is not so sensational as to prove embarrassing to the institution with which she is connected. Then, too, nurses are actually professional people, and one of the marks of membership in a profession is a certain breadth of vision and liberality of thought. Professionalism among nurses implies that they are *persons with ideas*, not only about nursing but also about public affairs, social and economic problems, in fact about all aspects of community and individual living which affect health. In order to develop this broad outlook, a nurse needs the same liberal education that any other professional man or woman receives before beginning to specialize.

Hence, it is our plan in the chapters which follow to encourage the nurse to feel at home in the whole realm of ideas. After engaging in a certain amount of ethical discussion, she should be prepared to think things through for herself, find out what it is that she really values in life, and use these values as principles to guide her in difficult situations that may arise later. All of this will be more obvious as we proceed with our discussion.

Study Questions

1. What do you consider the "proper business of an ethics course"?

2. Many centuries ago the Greek philospher, Socrates, posed the question: Can virtue be taught? Do you think that virtues, such as kindliness, sympathy, patience, and truthfulness, can be taught to nursing students if they do not possess them before entering a school of nursing? Should nursing schools take these virtues for granted and confine themselves to imparting knowledge and technics, or not?

3. Is it true in your own case that you would not want to be known as a highly moral person? Does the word "moral" have both a good and a bad connotation? What are the different meanings of the word?

4. Mention some acts that are commonly regarded as immoral which you think are harmless. Are there any acts which are considered moral by most people which you would regard as injurious to the individual or community?

Questions for Thought and Discussion

1. Do you think that each individual nurse ought to work out her own moral code? Should she receive her moral code from someone else? If so, from whom?

2. Do you think it would be possible for a hospital to set up rules and regulations which would prescribe the proper conduct for all the situations which might arise?

3. Do you think it would be possible for the instructors in a school of nursing to teach the correct behavior for every type of nursing situation so that students would have no conflicts about professional practice?

4. In a hospital ward, if there were a graduate nurse in charge for twenty-four hours of the day, would an occasion ever arise in which a nurse student would have to make her own choice between two possible courses of action? Give examples of the types of decision a nurse student has to make.

5. Do you think it would be desirable to have an official code of ethics for the nursing profession? Who would promulgate such a code? Would it be a compromise between conservatives and liberals, satisfactory to both? to neither? Would it contain concessions to strong minority pressure-groups? Who would interpret it?

6. Compare nurses with other professional people in regard to their leadership in public affairs. Do you know of any nurses who have been leaders in important modern social movements? What is the name of the nurse who was most influential in promoting birth control, or

planned parenthood, in this country? Can you name any nurse who has taught the medical profession a new method of treating a disease?

Books to Read

Dewey, John: *How We Think.* New York. D. C. Heath. 1933; Chap. I, II.

Landis, Benson Y.: *Professional .Codes* (Contribution to Education, No. 267) Teachers College, Columbia University, 1927.

VIII

The Harm That Taboo Morality Can Do

An unbiased view of anything often discloses both bad and good about it. Before we can turn to the constructive task of discovering rational principles of ethics for ourselves, it will be necessary first to get clear on one point: *not all moralities are equally beneficial to humanity.* Few people reach adult years without noticing about them a certain type of person, often in a position of leadership in the community, who is very sincere in thinking certain things are wrong, and often very devout in carrying out certain duties, but the things he thinks are wrong may actually be harmless and the things he thinks are right may be positively injurious to society. He is morally sincere but has mistaken ideas about what is right and wrong.

The standard by which our age measures any system of ethical belief is whether or not it is beneficial to humanity. Keeping in mind this standard, let us look at some injurious customs and beliefs in the world—not uncharitably, to cavil at the weakness or ignorance of others, but as objectively as possible. Instances from some distance away will be cited first as they illustrate the effects of an unthinking taboo morality more clearly than anything closer to us.

The Force of Taboos. There have been some primitive tribes, for example, in which it was considered the moral and religious duty of children to kill their parents when they reached an advanced age. This may have been necessary among some nomadic peoples who could take with them only those who were strong enough to ride a horse or camel. They naturally did not wish to leave to a death of slow starvation those who were weak. However, the practice continued in many tribes long after the origin of the custom had been forgotten and it was no longer a practical necessity. So we should say that it was

81

a bad, indeed a horrible, thing to do. And yet in the mind of
the man who put his parents to death the feeling of performing
a religious duty and obeying his conscience was very strong,
His conscience would have hurt him if he had *not* killed his
parents. Again, in several tribes of American Indians it was
considered a terrible sin for a man to speak to his mother-in-
law. He would have felt that it was a shameful, unheard-of
thing to do. If a traveler asked him why it was wrong, he could
only reply, "How could I talk to the woman who suckled my
wife as a babe?" This makes no sense whatsoever to us and
yet it is apparent that the Indian experiences the strongest
moral feelings in living up to this irrational taboo which he has
inherited from the past.

In the study of various cultures throughout the world there
are thousands of other examples in which tremendous moral
force and energy have been expended in enforcing taboos
having little or no relation to human welfare. Here is a list of
just a few things that we would say are harmless or even good
but which have been considered wrong by some peoples:

A man eating food touched by a woman.
Husband and wife eating together.
Man entering a tent pitched by a woman before it has been
"fumigated."
Woman speaking to a man who is on his way to war.
Woman crossing over into part of village set aside for
men's clubhouse.
Menstruating woman coming closer than a half mile to
a village.
Killing any animal.
Eating meat.
Reaching puberty without being married.
Being the mother of a man who has died.
Associating with persons of another caste.
Wearing shoes in a temple.
Wearing a low-necked dress.
Being seen without a lip ornament.
Woman uncovering face before anyone except husband.
Bearing a child without being purified for a month or more.

Woman appearing in public unaccompanied by a servant.
Saving a drowning person.
Failing to cook and eat, with appropriate religious cere-
monies, any person rescued from a shipwreck.

One of the saddest chapters in human history is the story of
the useless misery and death that have been involved in the enforcement of these and many other foolish taboos. Yet many of
the persons who for thousands of years have insisted on the
strict observance of such moral codes have been considered
good people in that they were sincere and conscientious. This
simply shows that it is not enough to be sincerely devoted to
what one thinks is right. One must also have an enlightened
conception of what is right. Otherwise one's goodness will
bring only unhappiness.

Illustrations from the History of Medicine

Exposing the Body. One of the traditions most closely identified with morality in our culture has been the taboo on exposure
of the body. Whatever rational justification may be given for
certain rules of decency, these rules were for generations
twisted into a narrow prudery that interfered tragically with
the practice of medicine. Only two or three centuries ago it
would have been considered scandalous for a physician to be
present during the birth of a child. Instead, only midwives were
called in. The first obstetrical work of any importance published
since ancient times, *The Garden of Roses for Pregnant Women
and for Midwives,* was written by a man, Eucharias Roslin, who
had probably never witnessed the birth of a baby! One of his
contemporaries, Dr. Werth, was burned to death in Hamburg
in 1522 as punishment for dressing up like a woman in order to
be able to study the several stages of labor.

It was not until the latter part of the seventeenth century that
men physicians were summoned in a few obstetrical cases by
royalty and members of the nobility. This innovation was then
gradually accepted by the common people. Opposition to it,
however, did not entirely cease until after the middle of the
nineteenth century. And during the intervening years many
women, who had got over being shocked at the "indelicacy"

of bearing a child in the presence of a man, still insisted that physicians should operate blind, with their hands underneath a sheet which covered the patient's body. Here is as clear a case as we can find where good, sincere people held traditional ideas about modesty and decency which hampered medical progress and efficiency and cost we know not how many lives.

Anti-Dissection. Other mistaken attitudes as to right and wrong have been equally unfortunate in their effects upon medical science. For many centuries it was considered wrong to dissect the human body and, even after dissections came to be permitted in the latter part of the Middle Ages, they were very rare and were permitted only on the bodies of executed criminals. As a result of this taboo on dissection, anatomy and surgery advanced very slowly and instruction in medical schools was even worse than it might have been. In fact, so great was the need for bodies in anatomical instruction that "body-snatching" became very common, and many persons, like Jerry Cruncher in Dickens' *Tale of Two Cities*, earned a living by stealing freshly buried corpses out of graveyards for sale to medical schools. Finally, after a series of notorious murders to obtain bodies, laws were passed in Great Britain in the nineteenth century making provision for the acquisition and dissection of bodies of persons other than criminals. Similar laws have been passed elsewhere. But this was a tardy victory of science over prejudice.

Anti-Vaccination. Another clash between unenlightened morals and medicine occurred when Edward Jenner, an English country physician, discovered vaccination for smallpox in 1798. He published an account of his investigations which showed that a harmless rash, called cowpox, immunized milkmaids against smallpox. His method of vaccination was derived from this discovery. Dr. Howard W. Haggard, in *Devils, Drugs, and Doctors*, says in connection with a reprint of the title page of Jenner's work, "The application of the facts presented in this paper has probably saved more lives than the total of all lives lost in war."*

* P. 230. Published by Harpers and Bros., 1929. Now in Blue Ribbon Books reprint.

If this is so, then opposition to vaccination is tantamount to dooming many persons to premature death who would have been saved by vaccination. Yet opposition began in the very year in which Jenner published his book. Anti-vaccination leagues were formed, which have persisted even down to the present day. But how can anyone in his senses oppose vaccination, when statistics show conclusively that where vaccination is enforced smallpox practically disappears? Today opposition is chiefly the product of ignorance and the machinations of non-medical healing cults. But originally not only ignorance but misguided moral and religious feeling was responsible. Many good people thought that it was impious to use artificial means to interfere with God's will. Since He had visited smallpox upon us in punishment for our sins, it was an affront to His will to try to save mankind from this affliction. Of course, if this logic were applied to every evil of life, we should have to abandon all our civilization. Building houses and hospitals, curing diseases of all sorts, performing the miracles of surgery, bathing, wearing clothes, using artificial light and heat, riding in automobiles, learning to read and write, are all directed against evils and thus the greatest accomplishments of modern man might be considered contrary to nature—a defiance of God's decree that we suffer for the sins of Adam and Eve.

Anesthesia. To us today it appears strange that human beings should be punished for the sins of previous generations, whether these sins were real or imaginary. But many good and other-wise kindly people in the middle of the last century opposed the use of anesthetics to ease the pains of childbirth on the ground that when God drove Adam and Eve out of the Garden of Eden, he put a curse upon Eve: "In sorrow thou shalt bring forth children." Hence, to reduce labor pains would be a wicked attempt to counteract God's curse. Not only many ministers and the lay public, but also physicians opposed the use of anesthetics. Fortunately, however, there were some surgeons, such as Sir James Simpson of Scotland, who struggled against this misguided piety. He was able to marshall both scientific and theological arguments in favor of anesthesia, one of the best of the latter being his rejoinder that God himself made the first use of an anesthetic, for when he created Eve out of one

of Adam's ribs he "caused a deep sleep to fall upon Adam."
This controversy, however, delayed the general adoption of
anesthesia a half century. Ether was first used in making operations painless by several American physicians and dentists
around the year 1844 but during the Civil War legs had to be
amputated without anesthesia and it was only at the close of
the century that the use of anesthetics became general. Science,
as usual, triumphed in the end, but what a pity that the service
which it offered mankind had to be delayed for many years by
sincere people!

Conservatism and Quackery. Sometimes misguided moral
ardor does harm by being attached to conservative practices
within the medical profession itself. One can be deeply, though
unintelligently, devoted to the good old way of doing things
or one can dismiss with a gesture of moral superiority any
discoveries made by outsiders. For example, Pasteur's discovery
that micro-organisms cause disease and his method of immuniz-
ing persons bitten by mad dogs were rejected by many medical
men who were suspicious of the experiments of a mere chemist.
They were righteous in their indignation against what they
regarded as an imposture but they were not wise enough to
recognize a new and revolutionary development in medical
science.

This sort of thing does not happen so often today, for the
method of scientific research is now well known and has become
thoroughly established, so that a properly conducted experiment performed by anyone, regardless of his professional label,
is usually accorded fair treatment. Non-medical healers, who
claim that their discoveries are arbitrarily suppressed by a
jealous medical monopoly, really receive little hearing because
they do not meet the most elementary requirements of scientific
research. Many of these people are sincere but science demands
much more than sincerity. Quackery can be conscientious but
still do as much harm, and even cause as much needless loss of
life, as if it were deliberately crooked.

Anti-Vivisection. Mention of quackery suggests another illustration of the unfortunate exercise of moral zeal—anti-
vivisectionism, which, though a lay movement, is often secretly
fostered by non-medical healers who want to throw as many

obstacles in the way of scientific medicine as possible. All of us share the sentiments which honest anti-vivisectionists feel about the suffering of dogs and other animals, but kindness loses its value when it is unintelligent. Anti-vivisectionist sentiment is unintelligent, first, because it fails to note that sympathy for dogs may be at the expense of thousands of human lives which might be saved by animal experimentation. Secondly, anti-vivisectionists are misinformed about the amount which dogs suffer. Anesthetics are used in operations on dogs just as on men. As Dr. A. J. Carlson of the University of Chicago said in a radio address at the Century of Progress Exposition in 1934, an animal suffering acutely would not be a fit subject for experimentation. He adds, "There is inflicted on animals more pain in one hunting, trapping, and fishing season than in all the centuries of animal experimentation." (One of the most famous anti-vivisectionists in this country has been noted for the expensive furs that she wears!) Dr. Carlson goes on to say:

"Free and intelligent experiments on animals during the last three hundred years have been the greatest factor in our present achievements in knowledge of life and control of disease. It was not till the great William Harvey began to observe and experiment on animals that we started to understand the heart, the blood, the circulation. We began to make real progress in the understanding, if not in the control of cancer, when this malady was discovered in animals and experimentally produced in animals. The lowly mouse, not to mention many other species, has served man well in research on cancer. Animal experimentation has been a great factor also in giving us better knowledge of anemia, digestive and kidney disorders, glandular disturbances, nervous diseases, the control of hookworm, scurvy, etc. There were more than thirty years of intensive research on animals—mainly on the dog—before we had the substance *insulin* in sufficient purity to warrant its trial on people sick with diabetes; and even now every new lot of insulin must be tested on animals before it is safe for the sick man, the sick woman, or the sick child. I sincerely believe that if every man and woman in this country knew the inspiring story of the discovery of insulin, all voices would be raised in approbation of such fruitful biological experimentation."

An even more striking illustration of unintelligent sympathy for animals is the Hindu doctrine of *ahimsa*, or non-violence, which prohibits one from killing any animal. Even mosquitoes are not killed by orthodox Hindus but are caught in a net at night and gently released the next morning. And rats, which carry the bubonic plague (the Black Death of the Middle Ages), are unmolested. Here we have a taboo which, by its forbidding direct violence against rats, makes inevitable the death of many persons in India and constitutes a threat against our own health, for without the strictest supervision of ships from the Orient, rats may come ashore and spread the disease here.

Venereal Disease. A last example of the way in which taboo morality can hamper medical progress is to be found in our own culture—our sexual prudery, which has long interfered with the prevention and treatment of venereal diseases. Science has done its part in discovering methods of preventing and curing these diseases, and it would seem that they ought to be most easily eliminated because we know specifically how the infections are transmitted. But our age-old prejudice against mentioning anything connected with sex has prevented us from giving the public the information it needs concerning the symptoms of syphilis and gonorrhea and the importance of immediate and consistent treatment by a regular physician instead of depending upon some quack or drugstore clerk for a remedy. Only in the past decade or so has the word "syphilis" appeared in print in American newspapers and it has been difficult for public health authorities to obtain permission to give frank talks over the radio about venereal disease.

A comparison of the prevalence of syphilis in Sweden and in Illinois will bring home to us the difference in human life and health which an enlightened public policy makes. And an enlightened public policy comes only after people shake off their prejudices enough to permit them to discuss freely all matters of health whether they are related to sex or not. In Sweden it is a criminal offense not to report a venereal disease or not to seek treatment either from a private physician or at a free public clinic provided for this purpose. The result is that the incidence of new cases of syphilis was less than 500 a year in Sweden in 1936 whereas in Illinois, which has about the same population, the incidence was about 14,600. No one is likely to claim that this difference can be accounted for by a difference in sexual promiscuity. Rather, it simply shows how intelligence combined with morality can produce health and happiness while unintelligent dependence on traditional moral taboos gets us nowhere in the solution of our problems.

The Waste of Moral Energy

The matters we have been discussing have been serious ones involving tremendous cost to humanity, and they illustrate taboo morality at its worst. People, good or otherwise, whose consciences function on the basis of such morality do harm to themselves and others by not becoming enlightened about the code which they inherit and blindly apply. Sometimes, however, the harm is not so serious, but shows itself merely as a waste of valuable moral energy. Keeping our objective point of view, let us complete our picture of mistaken moral ardor by noting some of these wastes.

Our Puritan Tradition. A generation or two ago the Puritan system, admittedly strong and beneficent at the time of the founding of this country, had disintegrated, some of its tenets passing over into the national philosophy, others, outmoded and useless, persisting in what came to be called Puritanical attitudes. They were a burden on our culture because they wasted moral energy that might much better have been devoted to things that really count for human happiness. They concerned questions of personal conduct such as card-playing, dancing, modes of dress, and even the length of women's hair—things most people regard as trivial and unimportant.

It is hard for many of us today to see how things like card-playing or dancing could have been or can be moral issues, or that people could have ever felt so keenly about them that membership in a church was denied to a person guilty of such wayward conduct. Yet this happened in some places two generations ago, and even as late as the time of the first World

War high school students signed cards pledging themselves never to dance. In the period after that war, however, there was widespread revolt against rules of conduct that could not be rationally justified in terms of human happiness. And no one seemed able to show how dancing reduced the happiness of either the individual himself or other persons.

Hardly credible to us also is the storm of protest that was raised against women's wearing knickerbockers. That, however, was just the beginning. Women who braved that storm were pioneers clearing the way for their sisters of a later decade who donned slacks or shorts with hardly a ripple of excitement in the moral community. Much moral energy was also expended in denouncing the younger generation for wearing short skirts and bobbing their hair, but ere long even the grandmothers were following suit. The intensity of feeling that was aroused, however, when women first began bobbing their hair can be seen from the fact that some employers threatened to discharge any girls who would be so "unladylike" as to have their hair cut and there were cases in which students were dismissed from schools of nursing for this offense.

While any one of these things in itself is certainly trivial, nevertheless all of them together form a part of larger trends which are of great importance and are fortunately in the right direction. One of these trends, which has been developing over hundreds of years, is the equality of the sexes. There are other trends also which will work out for the ultimate happiness of both women and men. But it is characteristic of traditional, taboo-morality that it is not aware of these developments but is capable only of blindly resisting everything new and different. On the other hand an ethics that is grounded on some larger principle of human welfare and an intelligent appreciation of the forces of history does not oppose desirable trends but welcomes any innovations that happen to be a part of the "wave of the future." Thus, as regards women's smoking, it may seem rather foolish for women to seek equality with men by adopting a habit such as cigarette smoking, yet the significant aspect of this for the moralist is the general movement toward equality. And he may also welcome the lifting of the taboo on women's smoking as one more contribution to the wholesome trend of placing more and more of conduct in the realm of taste or personal preference instead of in the realm of morals. But the main point to be noted is that all this opposition to things in themselves trivial has used up stores of moral energy, which, conserved for some really important public matter, could have wrought much good for humanity.

Unhappiness Caused by Sex Taboos

From time immemorial down to the present day there has been a great toll of women's lives lost for the simple reason that men and women lacked a knowledge of the reproductive processes and the means of controlling conception. This was unavoidable before the nineteenth century, but since then there has been in existence some knowledge of the means of preventing undesirable pregnancies and in the present century very scientific methods of controlling births have been developed by the medical profession. But for many years our policy of throwing a veil of silence around sex made us feel that it was improper even to discuss planned parenthood. As late as 1915 in New York City the police interfered with public meetings in which merely the question of the desirability of birth control was debated. In the meantime thousands of overburdened mothers were bearing an excessive number of children, growing more debilitated each year, finding it difficult to feed those already born, yet knowing that still others would be born. Some women, unable to endure the prospect of further pregnancies and knowing no means of preventing these, resorted to abortion, running the risk of death or invalidism resulting from inexpert or insanitary treatment at the hands of an untrained midwife or irregular physician. Others, using some sort of method of preventing conception, but with no scientific assurance of its reliability, suffered continual anxiety, so that the physical side of marriage was ruined for themselves and their husbands.

Birth Control. The past quarter of a century has brought remarkable progress in our attitude toward planned parenthood. Today, discussion of the subject is considered respectable in mixed groups, and a large section of the public is agreed on the desirability of having children only when they are planned for. There are now over five hundred birth control centers legally operating throughout the United States, and more and more private physicians are willing to give women and men who come to them scientific information about the control of conception. Even so, there are thousands every year who continue to have children in much the same accidental fashion as did previous generations, for we are still so much afraid of the subject of sex that most young persons are allowed to pick up information or misinformation as best they may rather than being given complete scientific information, including a knowledge of birth control.

At least partly as a result of this condition, there are probably more than 400,000 illegal abortions performed in this country every year, with several thousand deaths and considerable invalidism resulting. And it is a fact little suspected by the general public that 90 per cent of these abortions are had by married mothers, many of whom have already borne large families of children and know no other means of putting an end to childbearing.*

Then there are many mothers who bear children at the risk of their own lives and health. An element of taboo seems to remain in our morality when it has not yet become sufficiently enlightened to permit the public policy of teaching every woman how to have children only when common sense indicates that it would be good for her or the child. Instead a considerable proportion of the deaths that occur in childbearing are cases in which a physician could have told the woman that she would risk her life in becoming pregnant; or even cases in which a physician actually did warn a mother against another pregnancy but did nothing to provide the means to insure her against this danger.

Our traditional morality also still leaves us complacent about the fact that children continue to be born into homes where there is not enough money to give them proper nourishment and care. On the basis of intelligent planning we would see to it that, when the bread-winner is unemployed and a family is on relief, no more children are born. And all but a few irresponsible parents would agree that they should not bring

---

* See the study made by Dr. Frederick J. Taussig, *Abortion, Spontaneous and Induced — Medical and Social Aspects*. St. Louis. C. V. Mosby Company. 1936.

children into the world under such circumstances. Yet in 1932 the birth rate of families on relief was 54 per cent higher than that of families not on relief. But social workers still have to be very cautious about even referring these mothers to physicians and clinics for contraceptive advice.

Finally, there is one other class of cases in which pregnancy is unwanted or should be unwanted by the community. These are the cases in which either the husband or wife or both are feebleminded, or have some other hereditary defect. Here voluntary birth control is out of the question, the prohibition of marriage is futile in the absence of an adequate system of institutions for segregation and so the only feasible solution seems to be the sterilization of the feebleminded person. The laws of twenty-nine states provide for the sterilization of feeble-minded persons in state institutions but only in one state—California—has the law been applied extensively. In the others the law has been either inadequate or poorly enforced because of public and official indifference. Many people are ignorant of this danger to our social stock and the expense to the state in supporting defectives whether in or out of institutions. They are also uninformed of the nature of modern sterilization, which permits the person sterilized to have a normal sex life without the possibility of reproduction. This is due in part to the super-stitious awe with which we have shied away from the whole subject.

All of these evils would not exist in a world in which morality was directed toward encouraging knowledge instead of main-taining taboos on sex which produce widespread ignorance. The deaths, ill health, and lowering of racial stock which we have been discussing, however, are only part of the bad effects of our attitude toward sex. There are others which, while not so tangible and statistically demonstrable, are nevertheless just as real as far as human happiness is concerned. These are the maladjustments of marriage and of the period preceding marriage.

Segregation of the Sexes and Marital Maladjustments. There are two different ways in which our system of segregating the sexes produces unhappiness in marriage. One of them is the direct operation of segregation itself in reducing the opportunities for finding a compatible mate. The other is the indirect product of segregation which we have been discussing above— the feeling that sex is something immoral or not to be mentioned —resulting in ignorance of some of the things that are essential to satisfactory physical relations in marriage.

A conservative estimate might place the number of marital failures at around 30 or 40 per cent, if one does not have too high a standard of success.* In view of the fact that one sixth of all marriages in this country end in divorce and that some persons who would otherwise get a divorce are deterred by their religion, the proportion of divorces, were there no re- ligious pressure, would probably be one fifth or more. There are many marriages, too, in which economic necessity, the interests of children, or other factors, cause a couple to remain together even though their romance has turned to ashes and marriage can mean no more than practical cooperation in maintaining a home. Then, there are other couples whose marriage is not a complete failure but it may be highly unsatis- factory in some particular.

Now are we to blame such a large proportion of individuals for their marital incompatibilities? Are we to assume that they do not get along because they are too mean or selfish or fickle to make a success of marriage with anyone? That would indicate a very low appraisal of human nature. There are, to be sure, some persons who have characters that make them unfit for any permanent association with others but, if we think through the list of acquaintances of ours who have had difficulties in marriage, we shall find that the majority are persons who, apart from marriage, are agreeable, fairly unselfish, and constant in their affections. In their friendships within their own sex they frequently are highly successful without making any particular effort. Then what factor enters into marriage that is not present in friendship, to make for such a difference? Is it the sexual factor? It is true that this added adjustment accounts for some marital failures. But the principal difference is to be found in the way in which friendships and marriages are made. Friend-

* Sixty-three per cent of 526 couples reported their marriage as "happy" or "very happy" in the study by Burgess and Cottrell. (See *Predicting Success or Failure in Marriage*, p. 34. Prentice-Hall, Inc. 1939.)

ships are usually made easily and spontaneously out of a large number of casual acquaintanceships while marriages generally grow out of a very small number of social contacts with the opposite sex. Many persons in counting up would have to confess that they had selected a mate out of fewer real possibilities than could be numbered on one or two hands. Is it surprising that there are a great many incompatible marriages when they are based on such a limited range of choice?

The social conventions and moral attitudes, then, that tend to segregate boys and girls and make it much easier for them to form friendships within their own sex than with the opposite sex, are responsible for a large proportion of the failures in marriage. This segregation, however, to be understood must not be thought of in terms of strict rules, such as used to be employed in the patriarchal family in keeping women in seclusion. It is something more subtle. There is no law that prohibits social contacts between the sexes. But, especially in our urban civilization, there are conventions that make it relatively easy for men to form friendships with men or women with women. To make the same natural, easy approach to one of the opposite sex would be considered crude, boorish, "fresh." This attitude grows out of treating boys and girls differently from earliest years—dressing them differently, giving them different toys to play with, training them to have different ideals of life and conduct, providing different recreational groups for them—Boy Scouts, Girl Scouts, Y.M.C.A., Y.W.C.A., boys' classes and girls' classes at Sunday School, and so on. In some localities there are separate high schools and colleges for the two sexes and even in coeducational colleges the faculty and administration continue to follow blindly the old custom of building men's and women's dormitories at opposite ends of the campus instead of housing the two sexes near or even in the same building with a common lobby, dining room, and recreational rooms, as is done in the International Houses, established by the Rockefeller Foundation in a few of our big cities. When boys spend the greater part of their growing years with boys, and girls with girls, it is not surprising that all through life men easily gravitate toward men and women toward women, so that friendships within the same sex come with no effort while satisfactory associations with the opposite sex may be hard to achieve even with the greatest expenditure of thought about it.

Segregation continues also in our customs regarding appropriate occupations for men and women. For example, nearly all nurses are women, most doctors, dentists, engineers, and lawyers are men, women occupy most stenographic positions, and so forth. At the same time, in the modern city, neighborhood life has broken down and most of our social contacts grow out of occupational contacts. At work, however, men are mostly associated with men, and women with women, so that there is no escape here from the vicious circle which gives most people more contacts than they need within their own sex and not enough with the opposite sex.

Several generations ago the segregation of the sexes did not seriously interfere with the making of satisfactory marriages, first, because parents usually took the responsibility of marrying off their children, and second, because the ideal of marriage was simpler, since romantic love was not expected. Today, with our conception of marriage as a romantic companionship, we have a far more difficult ideal to realize. Yet our morality has not caught up with the new demands and does not provide the sort of social machinery that would give modern marriages a fair chance of being successful.

Political and Economic Ethics

We ordinarily do not think of ethics as extending to politics or economics, but the recent depression and war have brought home to us how persons and governments may devote themselves to ruinous public policies with all the zeal of moral reformers. For example, no one can doubt that there was moral fervor present in the brutal drive of the Nazis against the Jews. Not only leaders like Hitler but the rank and file of Nazis felt a glow of righteousness in the desire to make "pure" German blood dominant throughout the earth, with all other peoples serving merely as means to the ends of a German super-race. It is even possible to feel moral about deliberately breaking treaties or making promises with the full intent of breaking them as soon as convenient—all with the belief that any means is justified by the supreme end of national survival or supremacy. This sort of misguided morality has cost the lives of millions of people and the labor of years in building up productive capital.

On the other hand, the seeds of such fanaticism would have found little soil to grow in if we had not given ourselves up to a tradition of self-sufficiency. When knotty problems of economics presented themselves, it was easier to follow old paths than to face the risk and toil of blazing new ones. It is said, for instance, that two such mistakes were England's system of imperial preference by which she had the advantage over Germany in acquiring raw materials, and the American tariff wall which prevented Germany and other nations from sending us manufactured goods in exchange for our farm products and other commodities which they needed in order to enjoy a decent standard of living. Many persons in this country spoke with moral assurance about protecting American workers against the lower standard of living of European workers by maintaining a high tariff, when they had never really taken the trouble to think through the problem and find out whether our standard of living would actually be lowered or raised by more foreign trade. As a matter of fact, for years many eminent economists have favored a gradual lowering of tariffs. With greater production and exchange of goods, the peoples of other nations and also our own nation as a whole would be bound to have a higher level of living. Certainly the cost of war, which will never cease until all peoples have a fair chance to earn a living, is far greater than the temporary disadvantages that some classes of workers might suffer in a transition from high tariffs to free trade. One cannot solve these problems easily. But they must be solved. They can be solved by a morality that bids us obtain knowledge and use our intelligence to the utmost.

Role of Nurses. Nurses, ever since Florence Nightingale became immortal because of her work during and after the Crimean War, have been a blessing to wounded soldiers. And, of course, their first duty is to perform this sort of immediate service to suffering humanity. In the long run, however, a greater service can be performed by preventing the causes of such needless wreckage of human life by joining with other citizens in creating a better political and economic order in which wars will be impossible.

Similarly, in peacetime nurses do a service for which every person has occasion to be thankful at some time in his life. Yet the necessity for much of this nursing could be avoided if the economic problems of all people were solved so that they could have the medical care that would prevent much sickness, or if complete medical care came to be considered a human right to which everyone was entitled. Here again the nurse, along with other citizens, has a larger responsibility for using far-sighted intelligence in creating the sort of political and economic background in which preventive medicine will be most effective. Eventually this broader, social conception of moral responsibility may count even more for human happiness than the more obvious virtues which the nurse practices in her daily routine.

The Reconstruction of Morality

This chapter has been mostly of a negative character. We have seen how the mere fact that a person is conscientious and sincere is not enough. We must go farther and ask whether the morality that he or she is practicing is an intelligent one, productive of human happiness, or not.

John Ruskin said, "Follow your conscience but first be certain that it is not the conscience of an ass." Our business in the next chapter will be to work out some principles by which we may reconstruct our traditional morality in order to make sure that our consciences are doing good rather than harm to ourselves and others. This does not mean that *most* of our inherited morality needs to be revised. Quite the contrary. But where it does need revision, we ought to have clearly in mind some standard of judgment which we may apply with confidence and consistency.

Study Questions

1. Give several examples of sincere moral beliefs of primitive peoples which we regard as absurd.
2. Several moral attitudes which have hampered the progress of medicine are mentioned in the text. State each of

these in your own words in the form, "It is wrong to do so and so."

3. Enumerate some things that are now considered matters of private taste which were once regarded as violations of a moral code.

4. Make a list of medical evils resulting from the ignorance which is produced by the taboo on talk about sex.

5. Name two ways in which segregation of the sexes produces marital unhappiness.

6. How can nurses reduce disease and suffering apart from performing their regular professional duties?

Questions for Thought and Discussion

1. Some persons feel that, as long as one is sincere and devout in his beliefs, that is all that counts. On the other hand, we sometimes hear it said that any fool can be sincere. With which view would you agree? Is there some truth in both of these extremes?

2. If another nurse holds a moral belief which you regard as superstitious, would you rather she would *conscientiously* live up to her belief or would you rather she would be *unconscientious*, not take her morals or religion too seriously, and thus by ignoring her moral taboos agree in her actions with you? In other words, would you prefer *right motive* or *right behavior*, if you were forced to choose between them? Consider an example from the morality of Catholicism, Protestantism, Christian Science, Orthodox Judaism, Mohammedanism, or Cannibalism.

3. Have you set up for yourself some standards of conduct which differ from those you were taught in your childhood? If so, on what basis did you decide that new rules of conduct were superior to the old?

4. What would you consider a rational stand on the subject of women's smoking? Drinking? Do you favor a single standard of morality for men and women in all matters? In some things but not in others? If the latter, in what respects should their standards of conduct be different?

5. How far do you think we can go and ought to go in breaking down social barriers between the sexes? What are some ways in which you would suggest increasing social contacts between the sexes without going to the extreme of breaking down all barriers?

6. A middle-aged mother of a family comes to a free cancer clinic because of a lump in her breast. The doctor wishes to have his class of medical students examine the patient. The patient tells the nurse that she objects to having her body exposed to the view of these young men and that she will go home without being diagnosed and treated rather than submit to exposure. Are there other reasons than moral ones, why such a woman might refuse to be exposed? If you were the nurse in this situation, how would you try to convince this woman that she should allow herself to be examined and receive treatment?

7. In preparing a patient for examination or treatment, the nurse customarily "drapes" the patient. Is this draping chiefly to preserve the patient's modesty? What other reasons are there for covering patients with blankets or sheets during examinations or treatments?

8. A patient in the hospital is the mother of several children, none of whom has been vaccinated. The mother contends that no one in her family has ever been vaccinated and that none has had smallpox; she therefore sees no reason why her children should be vaccinated, especially as she fears it would disfigure their bodies with scars. Would you, as a nurse, feel any moral responsibility toward this situation? Would you try to convince the mother to have her children vaccinated? If so, what arguments would you use in favor of vaccination?

9. Ought vaccination for smallpox to be made compulsory?

10. Which is most effective in eliminating venereal disease: improvements in methods of cure, legal compulsion in regard to reporting and treating cases, legal control of prostitution, or moral suasion?

11. Do you know of any recent instances where medical

conservatism has prevented prompt acceptance of a new discovery?

12. In 1937, the American Medical Association at its annual convention recognized contraception (birth control by chemical, mechanical, or biological means) as a medical matter. Do you think that morality ought to pass judgment upon technics that are medically acceptable?

13. How would you solve the problem of reducing mortality and disability caused by illegally induced abortions?

14. Do you favor giving the government the power to sterilize the feebleminded? Certain types of criminals? If so, why? If not, why not? Do you think that a woman whose life will be endangered by pregnancy ought to be sterilized? Should a man be sterilized if he has a transmissible defect but is himself normal? Should a woman who can transmit hemophilia be sterilized?

15. What proportion of marriages in this country do you believe to be real failures? List some causes of marital unhappiness. Are there any maladjustments in marriage that are incurable? Would you favor the present law in your state specifying certain grounds for divorce or would you allow divorce to be granted on the ground of incompatibility? When a couple seeks a divorce because of incompatibility, what are some of the conventional charges used as a subterfuge under existing laws? Would you favor allowing judges to grant divorces after an informal conference without a court trial? What would be some of the advantages and disadvantages of such a system?

16. Do you think that political and economic attitudes should be treated as a part of our morality? Are these attitudes more important for human happiness than personal virtues or character?

17. Suppose that our economic problems were solved and everyone had a good living and could afford to pay for graduate nurse services, where would nurse students get their experience in taking care of patients?

18. What standard would you use in deciding whether a moral rule is good, bad, or indifferent?

Books to Read

Calverton, Victor Francis and Schmalhausen, S. D.: *Sex in Civilization*. Macaulay. 1929.

Crawley, Alfred Ernest: *The Mystic Rose; a study of Primitive Marriage*. New York. Macmillan. 1902.

Haggard, Howard Wilcox: *Devils, Drugs and Doctors*. New York. Harper. 1929. (Also in Blue Ribbon Series).

Mayo, Katherine: *Mother India*. New York. Harcourt, Brace. 1927.

Mead, Margaret: *From the South Seas: Studies of Adolescence and Sex in Primitive Societies*. New York. Morrow. 1939.

IX

Principles of Morality

Moral Relativity. People used to believe that all anyone had to do to find out what was right was to consult his conscience. They thought that conscience was a faculty implanted within them whose "still, small voice" always told them infallibly what was right. We have seen enough of what mischief conscience can do to know that it is not infallible. And we have got some inkling of an idea of the many variations and contradictions in the commands which conscience has given to different peoples throughout the world. The kind of conscience a person has seems to depend on the group into which he is born.

That is a rather startling conclusion to reach. If one's ethics depends upon the culture in which he is reared, how is it different from etiquette or all sorts of customs which also are relative to the group in which one lives? If we do not take customs very seriously and do not hesitate to adopt new ones as we pass from group to group, why take morality seriously either? Why not change our ethics according to the group we happen to be thrown with? Why not say, "When in Rome, do as the Romans do" when it is a question of morality as well as when it is a question of custom? Since adhering to our own morality really means subjection to the influence of the group into which we happen to have been born, why would not subjection to another group with a different morality be just as logical?

Or we might, in a spirit of revolt, say, "Why be subject to any group at all? If morality is just a tradition that our parents and ancestors have carried down from primitive times and imposed upon us, why should we regard it as sacred any more than we hold sacred such superstitions as its being unlucky for a black cat to cross our path? If morality is just the will of others implanted in us under the disguise of "conscience," why not assert our own wills and do what we please, since if it is a choice of wills we should naturally prefer our own?"

This skeptical attitude toward all morality is something that comes to every people that reaches the stage at which it can reflect about the origin of morality and its contradictions throughout the earth. Certain Greek philosophers, five centuries before Christ (the Sophists), had reached this stage and expressed their moral sophistication in the slogan "morality is custom," from which some of them concluded that morality deserved no more respect than custom and that a man was a fool to be held back by morality except in so far as he had to, in order to "get by" in a custom-bound society. An intelligent person, they said, would rise above the morality of the common herd and emancipate himself from slavish submission to tradition. For, after all, they reasoned, morality was just a device by which the weak members of society put pressure upon strong, self-assertive individuals to keep them under control. A strong man would be foolish to be taken in by that trick and meekly allow his conscience to deprive him of some of the choice pleasures of life.

Some college students today, after they have taken courses in sociology or anthropology or philosophy and learned that morality is as relative and variable as custom, also reason along the same lines as these Greek philosophers. They conclude that, since there is nothing sacred about morality and there is no way of showing that one group's conception of right is any more right than another group's, they will take the matter into their own hands and set up their own morality, which will be: "I'm going to look out for No. 1." Everyone for himself and let the Devil take the hindmost!

When these students are pinned down in an argument, however, they are usually unwilling to accept the full implications of their new "morality." They *do* care what happens to other persons and not merely about themselves. But their jumping to a conclusion of crass egoism shows how disintegrating the effect of moral sophistication can be.

Moral Emancipation. Even small children sometimes become aware of the fact that the voice of conscience is nothing but the voice of their parents keeping them under control. One mother was explaining to her four-year-old boy what conscience was. She said it was a little voice inside him which would tell him when he ought not to do anything. But he replied, "Aw, that's nothing but me remembering what you told me." This discovery that conscience is just the memory of what someone else has told us to do or not to do is harmless enough for a small child who accepts the authority of his parents. But for adolescents or adults the notion that conscience is an attitude implanted in us by others makes it appear an arbitrary imposition and we are likely to rebel and refuse to be bound by a morality which through a psychological trick enslaves us to the will of others. If we resent this imposition of the will of society upon us, we may decide to become "supermen" and throw off the yoke of authority, rising superior to the "slave-morality" of ordinary, unthinking people.

How about this? Is this a reasonable thing for an educated, enlightened person to do? Certainly we have subscribed in the preceding chapter to the notion that we ought to become sufficiently emancipated from authority so that we can rise superior to the dogmatic elements in our traditional morality which will not bear critical examination. But what about the rest of morality—the beneficial parts of it? Is this also to be repudiated?

To a certain degree, yes. That is, in so far as morality is felt to be merely something external to us—a subjection of ourselves to others—then self-respect and a sense of independence and individuality will lead us to reject the claims it lays upon us. That will mean that henceforth we will do things because we ourselves *want* to do them and not merely because somebody has told us it is our duty to do them. Our lives will be governed by our own disciplined desires rather than by pressure from a blind sense of duty.

This is not to say to anyone: Do what you like. There are several safeguards against such anarchy.

Why Moral Emancipation Is Not Dangerous

Morality Second Nature. In the first place, the social pressures under which we all grow up are enough to mold our desires into very much the same pattern. Even when we emancipate ourselves rationally from the dominance of society, we find that some of society's teaching is ineradicable. Some attitudes have become second nature with us and we cannot desire things that do not fit in fairly well with the needs of others. A person of normal heredity and social environment assimilates enough of the point of view of others so that it is quite safe to let him follow his own desires. And if there are some who are so innately selfish and cruel or who have happened to have such poor training that moral emancipation only makes them more selfish and cruel, these persons are few compared to those whom sophistication leaves as socially minded as before.

Kindliness. A second reason why it is safe to free people from an unthinking awe of morality, is that most persons have enough of the milk of human kindness flowing through their veins that, even when they simply follow their own desires, they find themselves spontaneously doing good for others. There seems to be something akin to the parental instinct that makes us sympathize with other people and care what happens to them. So, when we become free, our altruistic impulses are just as likely to come to the fore as our selfish interests. In fact, in an emancipated person, one of the principal motives for discarding irrational taboos is the desire to save society from the needless suffering that these often entail. Such a person is freed to do more good rather than less for others.

The Social Element in Emancipated Morals. Finally, when one comes to understand the social origin of morality, he does not usually just abandon morality altogether and think only in terms of desire. Rather he continues to think in terms of duty, or moral obligation, but along *reconstructed*, more intelligent lines. In such moral reconstruction, of course, he has to consult his own experience and his own desires, but the social implications of morality, e.g., the feel of the word "ought," set certain limitations upon his reflections. If the word "morality" is to have any meaning, it must refer not to just any desire but to those desires that are tied up in some way with social experience. The philosopher Immanuel Kant expressed this essential social characteristic of morality by saying that an act cannot be considered a moral act unless one is willing to have everyone act in the same way. Our morality is made up of those desires which we are willing to have universalized. Kant called this principle of universality the *categorical imperative* and phrased it thus: "Act as if the maxim of thy action were to become by thy will a universal law of nature." This is somewhat similar to the Golden Rule: Do unto others as you would that others should do unto you. Or, putting it in a little different way, we may say that certain demands which we make upon others should be made impartially upon everyone, including ourselves. That is, do not demand of others what you would not demand of yourself, and do not play favorites and apply a rule to one person when you would not apply it to another.

This principle of universality, or moral impartiality, grows quite naturally out of our early social experience and training in childhood. When parents reprove children, they generally reprove all alike. Children readily come to appreciate this fact and very early abstract out of their training the principle that what is right for one is right for another. Even very small children are insistent about having the same rules applied to their brothers and sisters as to themselves, and they even expect their parents to live up to the rules they impose. They also learn to make a distinction between demands that arise from whims of their parents and those that have a certain regularity and orderliness about them and are expressed with a tone of authority which gives the impression that they represent something more than the mere will of the parent. Morality thus acquires the feel of something that transcends the individual and is true everywhere and for everyone alike.

Those desires, then, which we want to have universalized constitute our morality. When we expect others to agree with us in regard to any matter of conduct—when we demand the same thing of ourselves and others—we are in a moral frame of mind, whether we use the word "ought" or merely the word "desire" to express this attitude. Hence, when an emancipated person falls back upon his own desires for guidance in living his life, he finds that *some* of his desires do not seem like mere whims but they have a sort of social halo about them—a sense of social backing, the sense of authority; and he feels a missionary zeal in communicating them to others. These socialized desires make up the reconstructed morality of an enlightened person, whether he calls it a morality or not. And the persistent element of sociality in such desires ties the individual to his group even after he has freed himself from its external authority. He is bound to it in both a conservative and progressive way. His individual experience will not lead him too far from the group tradition when he reconstructs morality, and he will also feel the urge to convert the group to whatever new morality he has worked out for himself.

The upshot of all this is that we do not need to be concerned about the desires of an emancipated person being anarchic or too individualized so long as they are desires which have grown up within a social context. Any desires accompanied by a willingness to have them universalized may be called a morality, and the reconstructed morality of an independent thinker is as genuine and dependable a morality as any merely inherited system. But, having reached this conclusion, we are still far from having a set of moral principles which will enable us to solve specific problems of conduct. We merely know now what constitutes *a moral frame of mind*, whether in a conservative or liberal, in a savage or a civilized man: *the willingness to have one's attitudes become universal.* But we still have to ask ourselves which attitudes *we* would like to have universalized.

Choices Underlying Any Particular Morality

The knowledge of what constitutes a morality in general is called by philosophers *formal ethics.* It is obvious that formal ethics enables us to recognize morality as a social phenomenon anywhere throughout the world, but it does not give us any guidance as to the content of the particular morality that we shall adopt. Head-hunting is a part of the moral code of some savages, and a member of such a group if asked whether he would want everyone to practice head-hunting would say yes. Similarly semi-civilized persons who believe in blood-revenge (avenging the honor of one's own family by injuring some member of the aggressor's family), would want everyone to follow the same code of honor. A Japanese who believed in suicide as a part of a code of honor would expect everyone worthy of his respect to adopt the same code. We, on the other hand, would want a different sort of conduct to become universal. Doing unto others as you would have others do unto you still leaves open the question as to *what* you would like others to do to you. The Golden Rule, or the formal principle of universality, gives us the minimum essentials of morality but it does not provide any guide as to the specific rules that should govern our lives.

Choices. In order to work out a morality of our own we must make four basic choices and each individual must make his or her own choice on the basis of previous experience and outlook on life. Each one has to answer these questions:

1. Who shall be included within the pale of morality? i.e., to whom shall morality apply? To a small primitive group? To one nation? To one race? To only one sex? Or to all human beings alike? In other words, shall there be one standard for all humanity? Or one set of duties for one group and another set of attitudes toward outsiders?

2. What is the supreme end, or ends, that I should seek? Happiness? Honor? Inner peace? What is it that I should value above all else in life?

3. For whom should I seek this supreme value? For myself? For my family? For my nation? For all humanity? If I should seek it for all of these and there is a conflict in interest, whose interest should I value more?

4. What means or what moral rules will best attain the end that I seek for myself or others? And how should these rules be applied? Rigidly with no exception, or with exceptions under certain circumstances?

When we have answered these questions, we shall see that we have a *working morality*. Let us turn, therefore, to a consideration of the first of the fundamental choices that we must make.

Humanitarianism vs. Tribalism

In the earliest times the only persons toward whom men felt any obligation were those within a small, isolated tribe. After thousands of years, however, civilized human beings have come a long way toward thinking of themselves as one big family or brotherhood. We treat other races and nations, at least in some respects, as well as we do our own. This widening of the circle of sympathy and morality to include everyone on the earth has been brought about through social contacts growing out of war and commerce and has been accelerated by the great increase in the speed of transportation and communication in the last two centuries. When human beings come to know one another better and the fear of strangeness wears off, their sympathies expand and they begin to share their attitudes and knowledge with one another. We might even say that on an earth such as ours and with the similarities in appearance and mentality existing among all men, it is inevitable that the unit of group feeling and morality should eventually become the whole world. Indeed, we not only feel sympathy with all humanity today but we even extend these feelings to animals as well and treat them as kindly as possible.

This tendency to feel a sense of community with all humanity was observable four centuries before Christ in the attitude of Greek philosophers, such as Socrates who, when asked of what city he was a citizen, replied, "I am a citizen of the world." The Hebrew prophets also showed signs of breaking away from narrow tribalism. Isaiah foresaw international peace, saying, "They shall beat their swords into plowshares, and their spears into pruning hooks: nation shall not lift up sword against nation, neither shall they learn war any more." And Jesus later gave numerous expressions to internationalism, e.g., "Many shall come from the east and west, and shall sit down with Abraham and Isaac and Jacob, in the kingdom of heaven."

In the centuries which have intervened much progress has been made in the direction of humanitarianism, in spite of temporary set-backs such as World War II. Even the war, however, made us more aware of our sympathies with remote peoples, for we found ourselves watching the newspapers eagerly every day for an encouraging bit of news from Britain or France or Norway or Russia or China. This concern for other peoples can be accounted for in part because of being united in a fight against a common enemy, but the more enlightened look forward to the time when a permanent peace can be established which will provide for the needs of former enemy nations as well as others.

Tribalism. It takes a long time completely to rid ourselves of the primitive attitude which regards only a limited number of human beings as worthy of respect and sympathy. There are

some persons who do not feel any obligation to be kind to
Negroes or foreigners or Jews except in the case of some
accident or other emergency, when humanity usually pushes
group prejudice into the background. The American Red Cross
is a good example of an organization which knows no color
line nor caste nor creed in its services throughout the world.
Yet many, who are enthusiastic about the work of the Red
Cross at times of great catastrophe, relapse into tribalism in
ordinary times and do not feel a humanitarian impulse to treat
other races or nationalities as they themselves would like to
be treated. They apply the Golden Rule only within their own
race or nationality or economic class.

We can understand how humanitarianism grows only slowly,
if we remember that old habits do not easily give way to new
ones. We naturally expect to find many unenlightened persons
far behind the vanguard of civilization. In the period following
the first World War—the war to end war—we took it for
granted that the idea of a world society and eventually a world
government was in the ascendancy, so that no great leader
ever again would have the effrontery to set up tribalism as a
moral ideal. In this we were mistaken, for first Mussolini and
then Hitler repudiated internationalism and humanitarianism.
Mussolini, for example, wrote in his article on Fascism in the
Italian Encyclopedia:

> Fascism does not, generally speaking, believe in the
> possibility or utility of perpetual peace. . . . War alone
> keys up all human energies to their maximum tension and
> sets the seal of nobility on those peoples who have the
> courage to face it. All other tests are substitutes which
> never place a man face to face with himself before the
> alternative of life or death. Therefore all doctrines which
> postulate peace at all costs are incompatible with Fascism.
> Equally foreign to the spirit of Fascism—even if accepted
> as useful in meeting special political situations—are all
> internationalistic or League superstructures which, as
> history shows, crumble to the ground whenever the heart
> of nations is deeply stirred by sentimental, idealistic or
> practical considerations.

Hitler went farther. Not only did he set up the Nazis as the only group worthy of respect and fair treatment, but he treated Jews and Poles as less than men. If he had had his way, all human beings would have come to be mere means to the end of Nazi glory and power. Rauschning quotes Hitler as giving the following description of the future society:

> There will be a master-class, an historical class tempered by battle, and welded from the most varied elements. There will be a great hierarchy of party members. They will be the new middle class. And there will be the great mass of the anonymous, the serving collective, the eternally disfranchised, no matter whether they were once members of the old *bourgeoisie*, the big land-owning class, the working-class or the artisans. . . . But beneath them there will still be the class of subject alien races; we need not hesitate to call them the modern slave class. . . . We must put an end to what is known as universal education. . . . We must be consistent and allow the great mass of the lowest order the blessings of illiteracy.*

Some of Hitler's remarks reflect the writings of the philosopher Nietzsche, who lived a half century ago and preached the doctrine of the superman. "Not mankind, but superman is the goal," he said. He repudiated the notion that morality applies equally to all persons:

> Moral systems must be compelled first of all to bow before the gradations of rank; their presumption must be driven home to their conscience—until they thoroughly understand at last that it is *immoral* to say that "what is right for one is proper for another."

Nietzsche did not believe in a single moral standard for all humanity. He thought the Christian virtues of humility, patience, sympathy, and kindliness were all right for the slave class but that the master class should not be bound by the

---

* Herman Rauschning, *The Voice of Destruction,* pp. 41–43. Published by Putnam's Sons. New York. 1940.

ordinary rules of honesty and decency and pity but should be haughty, domineering, boastful, selfish, quarrelsome, brave, cruel, and warlike. He urged "supermen" not to shrink from using lesser men as mere means to their ends, calling Kant "that great Chinaman of Königsberg" because he had said that humanity should always be treated as an end, never as a means. What a contrast between the respect which the German Kant felt for all humanity and the contempt in which these later Germans—Nietzsche and Hitler—have held the great mass of men!

Of course, in a certain sense even Nietzsche and Mussolini and Hitler have included all humanity within the pale of morality since they have felt the need of justifying themselves before the whole world. But aside from that they have certainly not acted toward those outside their limited circle as if they were entitled to any moral consideration. In this they have tried to turn back the hands of the clock of progress.

A World Morality. Most of us, who have been brought up in a democratic tradition which emphasizes the worth and dignity of all men, will have no difficulty in choosing between this narrow tribalism and humanitarianism. *More and more we are coming to believe in a single standard of morality and sympathy for all men and women throughout the world.* And nurses especially will have no hesitancy about choosing the broader type of morality, since as a profession they have long stood for world-wide humanitarianism.

That, then, is the first principle we shall adopt which will enable us to distinguish our morality from that of less civilized peoples or from that of some members of civilized communities who still cling to primitive attitudes and have not yet learned to think in terms of a world society. Viewed in historical perspective this is a decision of great importance. Yet in another sense it is the bare beginning of a morality. It merely commits us to this: that, *whatever our morality is, we shall want it to be adopted by all human beings and applied impartially to everyone.* It does not tell us what we want everyone to do or enjoy. In other words, it does not give us any information about the *supreme end,* or objective, of our moral desires and efforts.

Study Questions

1. What is conscience? What chiefly determines our ideas about right and wrong?
2. If we reject traditional morality, does that imply that our morality should henceforth be: "I'm going to look out for No. 1!" Why?
3. When we come to understand the origin of our morality and are emancipated from blind obedience to it, why does this emancipation not lead to anti-social conduct?
4. What is the difference between (a) the desires which constitute the morality of an emancipated individual and (b) desires which represent mere taste or whim?
5. State the principle of morality which Kant called "the categorical imperative."
6. If everyone in the world adhered to the Golden Rule, would this result in everyone's developing the same specific rules of conduct?
7. What are the four choices which determine the specific character of the morality which one adopts?
8. What is the meaning of humanitarianism as contrasted with tribalism (or ethnocentrism)?
9. Give evidences of the survival of tribalism among ourselves, the Nazis, the Fascists, and the Japanese.

Questions for Thought and Discussion

1. If conscience grows out of the instinct of children to imitate their elders and win approval and avoid disapproval by adopting the attitudes of their elders, how do you account for the fact that conscience sometimes tells us to stand out against our group for the sake of our principles? ("Blessed are ye though men shall revile you." "I'd rather be right than president.") If our principles come from the group, how can our principles conflict with those of the group?
2. How does the individual modify the conscience which he inherits from the group? In what kind of society is the individual more likely to reconstruct the morality which he receives from his group: in a small, primitive, iso-

lated, homogeneous group? or in a large, modern, heterogeneous society, i.e. one consisting of many conflicting groups and having many contacts with outside cultures? How have geographical factors, war, slavery, and commerce contributed to independent thinking in morals as well as in other matters? What is the effect of modern inventions such as rapid transportation and communication, moving pictures, and the radio in dissolving old cultures and encouraging individual thinking? How does education make one critical of traditional morality?

3. If morality is always *somebody's* desire (either a particular group's or a particular individual's desire), and "there is nothing either good or bad, but thinking makes it so," should we conclude that one morality is just as right as another? Is there an absolute standard by which we can judge that one morality is better than another? Or would this "absolute" standard just be the standard of the particular person who is passing judgment? What standard do *you* use in judging the value of various moralities throughout the world?

4. If you have known persons who have been emancipated from traditional morality, have you found them to be more or less selfish than others? Or about the same? Does a college education make students less moral or more moral? Less socially-minded or more so?

5. Would you prefer to room with a nursing student who treats you well because she feels it is her moral duty to do so, or with a student who spontaneously treats you well because she is naturally kindly and likes to see others happy? Which of these would make the better nurse?

6. Kant believed that one could deduce from the categorical imperative the following: (a) it is wrong to tell a lie under any circumstances; (b) it is wrong to break a promise under any circumstances; (c) it is wrong to commit suicide under any circumstances. Do you think that these rules necessarily follow from his principle? Could a moral person will that it should be a universal

law that exceptions should be made to a good rule under certain circumstances?

7. Are democratic countries justified in trying to make the whole world democratic? Does humanitarian morality imply that if we think democracy is a good, then we should desire that good to be shared by all men? Is this true likewise of modern science and technology? Is it our duty to carry scientific medicine and nursing to other peoples, even though they may be satisfied with their supersititions? If we think women are happier when free and more or less equal with men, as among us, ought we to hope that this ideal will some time penetrate into Mohammedan countries, as it has in Turkey, for example?

Books to Read

Drake, Durant: *The New Morality*. New York. Macmillan Co. 1928.

Hobhouse, L. T.: *Morals in Evolution, a Study in Comparative Ethics*. New Ed. rev. New York. Henry Holt. 1915.

Leighton, Joseph: *Social Philosophies in Conflict*. New York. D. Appleton, Century. 1937.

Niebuhr, Reinhold: *Moral Man and Immoral Society*. New York. Scribner. 1936.

Rauschning, Herman: *The Voice of Destruction. Revolution of Nihilism*. New York. G. P. Putnam's Sons. 1940.

Summer, W. G.: *Folkways*. Boston. Ginn and Co. 1907.

X

Ideals of Life

What is it that we want, and want others to join us in wanting and achieving? That is the next basic moral question to be answered. There are many things which we desire for ourselves but we feel no urge to have others share these desires or back us up in our pursuit of them. These are *matters of taste,* as we say. But what do we desire, with a feeling or expectation of social agreement and support? Whatever this may be, it constitutes our *moral end* or our *moral ideal.* This moral end may refer to ourselves alone, as, for example, when we feel that we must look after our future health and well-being. Or it may refer to other people. That is, we want others to act in certain ways or to have certain enjoyments.

To enumerate all the particular moral ends that we seek for ourselves and others would be an impossible task and would give us no principle by which to resolve conflicts and solve new problems. What we need to do is to find some common element running through all our moral desires. What is it *in general* that we want ourselves and others to do or have?

There are several fairly well defined types of answer to this question. These really constitute five philosophies of life, which we shall lay before the reader, attempting to present each of them with accuracy and fairness.

1. The Stoic Ideal: Serene Living
2. The Heroic Ideal: Living Greatly
3. The Ideal of Good Living: the Satisfaction of All Basic Needs
4. The Ideal of Free Living: Maximum Opportunity to Satisfy Any Desires
5. The Christian Ideal

Moralities may also be grouped into two large classes. In one of these a well-rounded life is sought in which no basic, earthly need is permanently sacrificed. In the other, the sacrifice of commonsense, worldly interests is often considered the highest realization of the ideal.

Life Guided by Traditional Duties. Before beginning our discussion of these ideals, however, let us say a word about a life guided simply by traditional duties. Those who lead such a life can hardly be said to have a conscious ideal or philosophy. But they do represent a way of life which is important because still so frequently encountered. Uncritical persons accept simply as ends in themselves a bundle of duties which have been inculcated in them in childhood. These duties are not valued because they are means to some higher end. They are felt to be "right because they're right," and the ordinary person believes that he ought to carry them out "just because he ought." These traditional duties do include some broader generalities such as being kind to others or making others happy, but when there is a conflict between some specific duty and some more general duty, most traditionally minded people feel powerless to resolve the conflict. Usually there is a tug-of-war in which the stronger duty wins but one still feels somewhat conscience-stricken for not having made the other choice. Conflicts arise between duties such as truthfulness, honesty, and living up to contracts, and the duty of helping others. In a morality in which all these duties are subordinated to some higher end, it is possible to weigh them against one another and reason about them, and when we make a choice, we have the satisfaction of knowing that we have made the wisest choice under the circumstances. But a person who only knows that contradictory duties are tugging at him flounders about like a ship without a rudder.

Also it is more difficult to reason with a person whose morality consists of a bundle of highly specific, fixed ideas about right and wrong. A good illustration of this may be recalled from *Gone With the Wind* in the scene where Rhett Butler was allowing his little daughter to ride her pony like a boy instead of sideways in a "ladylike" fashion. The old Negro mammy looking on was scandalized at the sight of a girl riding "a-straddle in front of her pa wid her dress flyin' up." In the movie version,

in reply to the father's arguments, mammy could only repeat,
" 'Tain't fittin,' 'tain't fittin,' 'tain't fittin'!"

All of us have a little of that blind sort of moralizing left in
us even after we have become quite sophisticated. But if we
learn to bring our many independent rules of conduct under a
more general end, we can at least reason some of our irrational
taboos away. Let us proceed then to the examination of the
several ideals of life which offer themselves as guiding principles
in making our morality more rational.

The Stoic Ideal: Serene Living

Happiness, according to philosophies which sacrifice common-
sense, worldly interests, does not require a harmonious expression of *all* sides of human nature but may consist in devoting
oneself to *one* special end, or to a virtuous life narrowly defined,
at the expense of other interests. Renunciation, abstinence, discipline, and sacrifice are key words in this type of morality.
Stoicism is such an ideal, consenting as it does to sacrifice any
of even our fondes   _s for one supreme value—serenity.

The Ancient Sto.._. Stoicism originated in ancient Greece
several centuries before Christ in a period of decadent political
life and general insecurity. In fact, nearly all ancient philosophies and religions were based upon a sense of hopelessness
and pessimism regarding human affairs. There was no belief
in progress, such as we have today, for the Golden Age was
located in the remote past rather than the future. Everywhere
there was a sense of decline and decay and a feeling that no
one could do anything to change the world. Now when men come
generally to believe that "you can't do anything about" the
world, the only resort left is to resign oneself to things as they
are and concentrate on maintaining a calm, unperturbed state
of mind regardless of what happens.

So the Stoic philosophers told men not to let their happiness
hinge upon any worldly goods, such as property, honor, health,
or love, but only upon the things that are "within our power,"
i.e., upon inner adjustments of our desires, so that they always
conform to reality. If we set our heart upon nothing more than
the inner satisfaction of controlling our desires, maintaining
right motives, keeping our emotions on an even keel regardless

of external circumstances, then we can never be disappointed.
No one can take away such inner peace. They can throw you
into jail, the Stoics said, but they cannot keep you from wanting
to be there, or at least from being resigned to being there. As
the English poet, Lovelace, wrote:

> Stone walls do not a prison make
> Nor iron bars a cage.

If we can train ourselves to be indifferent to the buffets of
fortune, nothing can hurt us. We are invincible, said Epictetus,
the Roman Stoic:

> A good man is invincible; for he doth not contend where
> he is not superior. If you would have his land, take it; take
> his servants, take his public post, take his body. But you
> will never frustrate his desire, nor make him incur his
> aversion. He engages in no combat but what concerns the
> objects of his own choice. How can he fail then to be
> invincible?*

It is interesting to note that the two most famous Stoics of
antiquity were Marcus Aurelius, an emperor, and Epictetus, a
slave. If one's happiness depends only upon inner values, then
it does not matter whether one is an emperor or a slave. Though
a slave, one can be free and enjoy a sense of great power by
being in command of one's emotions and desires.

Happiness may be expressed by a fraction in which the numerator is what we have and the denominator is what we want,
so that if we have one thing and want two, our happiness fraction amounts to one-half or fifty per cent. Now we can bring
our happiness up to one hundred per cent either by adding to
what we have so that both the numerator and denominator become two or by subtracting from what we want so that the
numerator and the denominator become one. But which is the
surest way to win happiness? The Stoics believed that it was a
vain hope to seek to control the world and increase our external
goods. It is much simpler, they said, to control ourselves and
cut down on our desires until they equal what the world has to
offer us. "Require not things to happen as you wish, but wish

* *The Discourses of Epictetus*, p. 144, Everyman Edition.

them to happen as they do happen, and you will go on well."
According to this approach to life, a true Stoic should be happy
under even the most trying circumstances.

> Who, then, is a Stoic? Show me one who is sick, and
> happy; in danger, and happy; dying, and happy; exiled,
> and happy; disgraced, and happy. Show him to me, for,
> by heaven, I long to see a Stoic.*

The Stoics even went so far as to say that a man could be
happy under torture. By just looking upon pain—even our own
pain—as an interesting natural phenomenon, we can become
indifferent to it and rise above it. We know today that this is
true to some extent. A person who is on edge and expecting
to be hurt every minute suffers much more in the dentist's chair
than a person who is calm and relaxed and tries to detach
himself from the pain. But it stretches our credulity a little too
far to believe that anyone could ever adjust his desires enough
so as to be happy under torture. The Stoics, however, were
fond of relating the story of how the slave Epictetus behaved
when being punished by his master. When his leg was being
twisted, he remained perfectly calm and with a matter-of-fact
look on his face glanced down at his leg and said to the master,
"If you keep on twisting that leg, it will break." Surely enough
it did break, and Epictetus with equal calmness said, "See, I
told you it would break." That is carrying equanimity, or
imperturbable inner peace of mind, to an incredible extreme.

Inadequacy of the Stoic Philosophy. What can we say of this
philosophy? Most of us would say that it is impossible to adjust
our desires so as to make ourselves acquiesce in every misfortune that befalls us. Also, there is danger that, if we resign
ourselves too readily to external evils, no improvement will
be made in the world around us. Indeed, the world might go by
default into the hands of criminals who would have their way
entirely if most of us became resigned, non-resisting Stoics.
And, even if that were not true, the question might be asked
whether inner serenity is worth living for, if that is all we have
and if it is at the cost of renouncing most of the things we
naturally care about. It is a rather thin and pale kind of happi-

* *The Discourses of Epictetus*, p. 112, Everyman Edition.

ness, which avoids great desire and great risks in order to be
secure against disappointment. Most people would rather
gamble for big stakes and take the chance of losing and suffering
much. Irwin Edman has expressed well this preference for great
living, as against the drab security and mediocrity of Stoicism,
in his poem, *They Do Not Live:*

> They do not live who choose the middle way,
> Whom ecstasy and anguish have not known,
> Who scale no trembling heights nor plumb the lone
> Depths of an aching darkness in bright day.
> They miss the passion with the pain, the gay
> High tides that lift the spirit to its own,
> The lifting surge of music, the dear tone
> Of a loved voice in pleading or in play.
> They miss the hurts and stumblings; surely fear
> Is never theirs, nor groping in the night;
> In their serene cool weather come no dread
> Torrents or tempests to corrupt their sight,
> Nor any rainbow; neither do they fear
> The sea, nor does the thunder wake these dead.*

The Stoic ideal, then, does not offer a rich enough conception
of happiness to merit its adoption as a whole by a progressive
society. At the same time, as one phase of a broader view of
life, stoicism may stand us in good stead in time of trouble.
Sometimes we find ourselves up against a stone wall where
there is absolutely nothing we can do. Some accident of birth
or of experience may utterly shut us out from certain types of
satisfaction. In such cases we have the choice of becoming cynical
and bitter against life or of salvaging what we can of happiness
by resigning ourselves to the inevitable and making the most
of our other powers. This is the sort of stoicism that all of us
can subscribe to and which we have to make use of at one time
or another in our lives.

The Heroic Ideal: Living Greatly

Stoicism, as we have seen, is a sacrificial ideal. It does not
hesitate to sacrifice any or all worldly desires on the altar of

* From *Poems* by Irwin Edman. New York. Simon and Schuster. 1925.

its supreme value—equanimity. For it the attainment of a well-rounded life which satisfies the strongest human desires is not essential to true happiness. Happiness is to be won by learning to renounce the things that most people care about.

The Strenuous Life. A similar repudiation of happiness as many conceive it is found in the heroic ideal. In this the supreme end of human striving is not a peaceful, smooth-flowing, contented, harmonious life but a strenuous life in which all ordinary satisfactions may be risked or lost in overcoming some obstacle. It is the quality of striving, the zest of battle, the stress and strain of great endeavor that is valued above all things. It is *great* living as opposed to *good* living. What strikes the good liver as a foolish throwing away of life on a single enterprise is called by the advocate of great living a "magnificent obsession!"

Such an ideal was the motive force of the hero of a best-selling novel of a few years ago, *The Forty Days of Musa Dagh.* A young man of rank and wealth, native of a small European state who has lived a pleasant, aimless life, suddenly finds that his country is being invaded, and, gripped by a power he never dreamed he had, leads the people of his community in a successful forty-day stand against the conqueror. He feels an exultation that to him is the supreme value of life. At the end of the book, he returns to die in the ruins of the fort he held because death on the scene of that experience was worth more than life anywhere else.

Historic Examples. The heroic ideal has been expressed in various ways in the course of human history. Codes of honor, such as the dueling code which was accepted in the early days of our Republic or suicide for the sake of honor among the Japanese, are examples. In a dueling code it is supremely important to maintain one's honor by accepting all challenges. No matter how foolish the practice may be, no matter how unjust the challenge, no matter how unscrupulous the challenger (e.g., Aaron Burr against Alexander Hamilton), nevertheless honor requires that every other consideration be sacrificed. It is better to die nobly than to live ignobly, or even ordinarily, the supporters of this way of life argue.

The power and appeal of this system has been often demonstrated. Whatever we think of the results of the theories of Friedrich Nietzsche in our generation, we cannot deny their force. The superman of this German philosopher is a protagonist of the heroic ideal. He disdains the mild, gentle, humane virtues of the democrat and Christian. "What is good?" said Nietzsche. "To be brave is good. What is good? All that increases the feeling of power, the will to power, power itself, in man. What is bad? All that comes from weakness." "Zarathustra (a mythical character into whose mouth Nietzsche puts his doctrine of the superman) was fond of all such as make distant voyages, and like not to live without danger." "A good war halloweth any cause." Nietzsche admired the exciting, vigorous life of his cruel Teutonic ancestors more than the peaceful, industrial civilization that he identified with Christianity and democracy. They were, he says, "free from every social restraint; in the innocence of their wild-beast conscience they returned as exultant monsters from a horrible train of murder, incendiarism, rapine, torture, with an arrogance and compromise as if nothing but a student's freak had been perpetrated."*

Hitler's views reflect Nietzsche's glorification of hardness and contempt for the gentler virtues in one of his conversations recorded by Rauschning:

> In my great educative work I am beginning with the young. We older ones are used up. Yes, we are old already. We are rotten to the marrow. We have no unrestrained instincts left. We are cowardly and sentimental. We are bearing the burden of a humiliating past, and have in our blood the dull recollection of serfdom and servility. But my magnificent youngsters! Are there finer ones anywhere in the world? Look at these young men and boys! What material! With them I can make a new world.
>
> My teaching is hard. Weakness has to be knocked out of them. In my *Ordensburgen* a youth will grow up before which the world will shrink back. A violently active, dominating, intrepid, brutal youth— that is what I am after. Youth must be all those things. It must be indifferent to

---

* Quoted by Will Durant in the chapter on Friedrich Nietzsche in *The Story of Philosophy*. Garden City Publishing Co. Nietzsche does not recognize here that the democrat or Christian may be a militant crusader.

pain. There must be no weakness or tenderness in it.
I want to see once more in its eyes the gleam of pride and
independence of the beast of prey. Strong and handsome
must my young men be. I will have them fully trained in all
physical exercises. I intend to have an athletic youth—
that is the first and the chief thing. In this way I shall
eradicate the thousands of years of domestication. Then I
shall have in front of me the pure and noble natural material. With that I can create the new order.*

Mussolini also in his article in the Italian Encyclopedia, in-
corporated the heroic ideal into the Fascist philosophy. "Fascism," he said, "emphasizes the strenuous life. It rejects absolutely the idea of an easy life. The Fascist accepts and loves
life. . . . Life as he understands it means duty, elevation,
conquest; life must be lofty and full."

To what end was all this strenuous living? What did the
Italian people gain from it? These are questions that will be
asked by anyone who believes that the only happiness worth
striving for or sacrificing for is a well-rounded, harmonious,
peaceful life. To him the heroic life is a delusion, a piece of
arrant nonsense. Heroism, great deeds, and the martial spirit
have value, he would say, only when they are *necessary* in order
to create a world in which such living will no longer be urgent.
But those who value the life of great striving for its own sake
will not be impressed by such objections, for they will reply
that the satisfaction of living honorably and courageously is
greater by far than any of the humdrum, commonplace satisfactions of peace and plenty. Here we have an irreconcilable
difference as to what is ultimately desirable.

Good Living: the Satisfaction of All Basic Needs

The sacrificial ideals which we have been examining may
have had great value and may still have value in critical times.
They are useful when there are obstacles to overcome or when
there are obstacles which cannot be overcome. They tend,
however, to become ends in themselves. They have been so

* Hermann Rauschning, *The Voice of Destruction*, pp. 251–252. New York.
G. P. Putnam's Sons. 1940.

important at times in human history that they have come to be regarded by some as ultimate ideals, desirable in themselves and expressing the very essence of true happiness. This view, however, has been largely one of leaders, especially in war. It has never been wholeheartedly accepted by ordinary people. When they say they want to be happy, they mean that they would like to have a well-rounded life with a generous and fairly secure satisfaction of *all* their urgent desires. They want health, the esteem of their fellows, the affections and satisfactions of marriage, and a certain amount of excitement or recreation. They also want an opportunity to express the parental impulse either in the home or in the world at large where there are people who need their help, and they want to see the things done which they consider right and just.

Essential Satisfactions. In a word, happiness defined in this manner consists of:

1. Health
2. Social status
3. Intimate affection
4. Recreation
5. Parental feeling or sympathy
6. Rightness

The first four of these essentials represent primarily the receiving side of a happy life. They are the things we long to *enjoy*, though, of course, they do not consist merely of passive enjoyment but may involve much activity. In the other two essentials the stress is primarily upon the satisfaction of *doing* things, or getting things done. In a well integrated character, however, there can be much joy in these activities in which our principal concern is not what we are getting out of them for ourselves.

The Well-rounded Life. Not only has common sense always told most men and women that a life cannot really be called happy unless it contains all these satisfactions but also in the past century there has been a growing tendency for this fact to be recognized by moral philosophers as well. A group of moralists called Utilitarians have especially promoted this view of life, and others too, who have disagreed with the Utilitarians about some issues of merely academic importance, have sub-

scribed to the ideal of a well-rounded life, whether they have
called it "happiness" or "well-being" or "self-realization," or
what not. Apart from academic quibbles, the significant thing
about this modern view of life is that it regards no part of man's
nature, such as sex, for example, as essentially bad; the ideal
is to achieve a harmonious, wholesome satisfaction of all desires. A life which is unnecessarily filled with ascetic self-denial
and suppression of basic impulses is considered a warped life
rather than a good one. The moral ideal is that every human
being should enjoy an abundant life, rich in all the satisfactions
that men and women commonly seek.

Morality a Means to Human Happiness. Another significant
thing about this doctrine of well-rounded happiness as the end
of life is that all moral rules become subordinate to it. This
means that no part of a moral code is to be regarded as eternally
right. A moral rule is right only so long as it promotes the
general happiness. The Utilitarian view is that no virtue should
be practiced at the continued expense of human happiness, for
this implies that virtues are fixed and unchangeable and worth
more than all other satisfactions. Utilitarians hold that the
virtues which form the moral code are simply *means* to the larger
end of an all-around, satisfying life. They might paraphrase
Jesus' words that "the Sabbath was made for man, not man for
the Sabbath," and say that morality was made for man, not
man for morality. Human happiness should not be sacrified on
the altar of an inflexible morality but morality should be regarded as a social device by which happiness may be promoted.

This does not mean that morality as such may not be valued
for its own sake. Thus, we have listed "rightness," or the satisfaction of seeing justice and right prevail in the world, as a
basic need. The enjoyments of life, for most of us, would lose
their savor if we turned our backs on the world and did nothing
to make it better. Doing right is one of the essential values of
a happy life, and thus in the course of our training and experience it has evidently become an end in itself. But this is not the
same as saying that a *specific* set of virtues should become the
supreme end and never be subject to modification.

The ideal of a well-rounded life is the most inclusive of any
that we have studied and has a strong appeal to men and

women of the modern world. While not everyone can attain it in full, still the tendency today is to want to see as many people as possible enjoy such an abundant life. Circumstances may make it necessary for some of us all of the time and all of us some of the time to content ourselves with a life of resignation and inner peace instead of a lusty pursuit of external values. But the modern world is suspicious of any one who sets up his particular adjustment to misfortune as a positive, universal ideal. It is all right to make a virtue of necessity for ourselves in order to salvage what we can of happiness in times of adversity, but for humanity as a whole the ideal is the most complete happiness that each one can attain.

Free Living: the Maximum Opportunity to Satisfy Any Desires

The ideal of a well-rounded life leaves a great deal of latitude for the expression of individual taste in satisfying *each* of the basic needs. The only limitation upon individuality is the demand that no single desire should dominate our lives to the exclusion of other strong impulses. Those who hold the ideal of a well-rounded life cannot believe that people are really happy who lead a one-sided life or miss some of the basic satisfactions. On the other hand, some moralists believe that there is danger in thus passing judgment upon other people's mode of seeking happiness. No one knows so well as the individual himself what he really wants, they say, and it may be that a devotion to a narrow set of interests really gives some persons more satisfaction than a well-balanced life could. They go in for depth rather than breadth. At any rate it is argued that morality ought not to go back of the individual's report as to what he wants. Desires should be taken at their face value and morality should simply make it its business to see to it that *opportunities* are provided for the maximum satisfaction of all desires which can be satisfied in society, whether they be broad or narrow, wise or foolish, in the opinion of others. This is the doctrine of freedom, or *ethical individualism*, as it is sometimes called.

T. V. Smith lends eloquent support to this in his *Promise of American Politics:*

There are, as there have always been, men who believe themselves commissioned as custodians of other men's souls. Such men will not ordinarily admit of others (as they are certain to feel of themselves) the truth of our first plank (that there is no good independent of human desire). . . . Even if they admit the truth of our first contention, they will nevertheless seek to avoid it by distinguishing between what men "want" and what they "need," setting themselves up as dispensers of special light upon the latter.

Against all such, we set the simple belief that each man is the best judge of what he desires. Even if he "needs" something else, his need for it will not be adequately satisfied until he *wants* what he needs. Let it not be thought, however, that we are romantic as to the extent to which common men, or other men, understand themselves. We are not perfect judges of ourselves. Of our wants we are most ignorant. . . . Ignorance of our own nature and of the world stands in our way. We commit ourselves to what we thought we wanted, only to find later—often too late to rectify—that if we had known the consequences of what we thought we wanted, we should not have wanted it at all. Men really want only what they will continue to have wanted after the consequences are in and the bills are paid. . . .

No, few moderns know what they want. Wants are multiple in a world of competing goods. Every man is in some measure the hero who jumps on the horse of heavy desire and rides off in all directions at once. We find it next to impossible to make up our minds steadfastly as to what we want. But, if it be so difficult for each to know his own wants, is it the wise man or the wiseacre who thinks that he knows more about another's wants than that other knows about them?*

This ethical individualism, or the ideal of happiness freely defined, envisages a world in which everyone has the greatest opportunity to work out his salvation along the line or lines

* Pp. 82–84, University of Chicago Press, 1936.

that suit him. If he prefers a life of Stoic serenity, a strenuous life, or a well-balanced life—any of these will be all right from the standpoint of ethical individualism, if only the individual is successful in achieving his heart's desire and if he himself continues to assert that he really wants what he wants.

The Christian Ideal

When a system has the sweep of appeal geographically and historically that we associate with the Christian ideal, there is generally a reason for it that can be discerned on examination. It is so here. As we discuss it, there will appear an inclusiveness, a variety of appeal, a flexibility and possibility of multiple adaptation, that belongs to no other ideal. It has many facets. Almost everything under the sun has been given the name "Christian" at one time or other, and within Christendom there exist such varying codes that definition is far from the easy task offered by any of the previous ideals. Indeed, it may include features of each of these others. Strictly it is not a system in the sense that they are, but is distinguished by its capacity to hold and apply in its own way their varying appeals.

Christianity exhibits Stoic elements when it bids us rise superior to the buffets of fortune or the contempt of wicked men: "Blessed are ye though men shall revile you." It represents the heroic ideal of living greatly when it tells us to lose ourselves in something greater than ourselves: "He that loseth his life shall surely find it." The "more abundant life" of Christianity may be interpreted as equivalent to a well-rounded life and the Utilitarian emphasis upon consequences may be found in Jesus' saying, "By their fruits ye shall know them." And, finally, the ideal of free living finds some support in the tolerance and breadth of sympathy exhibited in many acts of Jesus and in his injunction: "Judge not that ye be not judged."

In addition to these elements found in other systems, there is one outstanding tenet on which all Christians are agreed, at least in theory, and that is the brotherhood of man. Christianity has been one of the foremost forces in the world promoting the humanitarianism which we affirmed at the close of the last chapter. Humanitarianism tells us that whatever morality we espouse must be applied to all human beings alike. Morality must know no boundaries of class or nation or race.

Christianity stands for kindness and mercy and love of one's neighbor. And when we ask, "Who is my neighbor?" it is clear now after many centuries that my neighbor means everyone in the world. So this aspect of Christianity is equivalent to the general principle of seeking the well-being or happiness of all humanity. Such a principle might well be used to unify and rationalize all moral rules. In deciding whether to adopt or reject a traditional maxim or taboo, we should simply ask: Does it produce human happiness or not? And eventually we should have a moral code every bit of which was beneficial to man and none of it harmful. Such a morality would appeal to every socially minded man and woman. Here we find Christianity marching with modern international trends and with the broadest views of ethics.

Christian Conception of Happiness. When we seek a definition of "well-being" or "happiness" in the Christian tradition, however, we find varying conceptions through the ages. Does happiness mean a well-rounded satisfying life here on earth or does it mean eternal bliss in some future heaven? Or both? If the happiness which we should seek for mankind is eternal salvation, does that mean we should be indifferent to earthly happiness? The answers to these questions establish the fact that certain phases of Christianity in history, notably the Puritan phase, have tended toward a sacrificial ideal. In these phases it would seem that the adaptation of Christianity has been made to periods which demanded sacrifice if the race was to progress. Thus the stern old Puritan Father, leaning his gun inside the door of the log church and settling himself in the freezing atmosphere for a two-hour sermon, may well have considered this life pretty much a vale of tears, and proceeded to cancel out the prospects of happiness in it as a dead loss, and to concentrate on strength of character and the life to come. This same old worthy no doubt also blacked out the pleasures of life for his numerous sons and daughters. As the new nation progressed, however, and times became happier, these children and their children nevertheless kept as their traditional morality some of the old admonitions and the result was the taboo type of morality discussed in Chapter VII.

On the other hand, in modern times there has been a growing number of Christians who have believed that the best way to deserve eternal life is to make human society here on earth as happy as possible. They have believed that progress is possible and that the world can be made a very pleasant place to live in, free from war and poverty and most of the sicknesses that have oppressed it in the past. Such a this-worldly attitude allies Christianity with the ideal of abundant living. Yet there still remains the problem of *defining* happiness. It has always been assumed in Christianity that God wills the happiness of his creatures. Difference arises in the methods by which Christians find out what happiness consists in.

Sources of Moral Wisdom. There are three larger classes into which Christians fall today as regards their solution of this problem. Some would say that if we wish to learn God's will and the kind of happiness he desires us to have and also the virtues necessary to achieve this, we should go to the Bible and read God's word there. This is the more conservative Protestant position. Others would say that God continues to reveal his will through the official utterances of Church author- ities so that both the Bible and the Living Church, but especially the latter, are the sources of our knowledge of true happiness and Christian morality. This is the Catholic position. The third group of Christians, who are generally referred to as liberals, believe that revelation of truth and right is not limited to Bible or church but occurs also when any intelligent and well-disposed person tries to find out what is true about the universe and what will produce the greatest happiness for man- kind. For the liberal, experimentation in scientific laboratories and careful investigations made by social scientists are the best modern sources of knowledge. He also believes that the shared experience and cooperative thinking of each succeeding genera- tion will bring us closer to wisdom in morals. If there is a conflict between moral rules prescribed by Bible or church and the conclusions reached by modern society regarding the moral code most conducive to happiness, the liberal believes in depending upon modern inspiration. He regards the Bible as a piece of ancient literature containing much wisdom but also many passages that have been found to be unsuited to the needs of modern society.

The liberal Christian view of morals is *in practice* exactly the same as that of anyone who believes in human happiness as the objective of morality and believes that it is the task of each generation to work out for itself experimentally the wisest rules for attaining happiness. And, in fact, in large segments of life in which no hard and fast rules have been laid down by Bible or Church, conservative Protestants and Catholics also take this experimental attitude. It is only in the part of morality where there are very specific prohibitions, such as those against remarriage after divorce, abortion, euthanasia, contraception, and sterilization that Christians part company with one another.

Christian Character. Probably the phase of Christian morals about which there is the most theoretical agreement but the least popular understanding, is the ideal of Christian character. Although it has included notable emphasis on vigor and courage, it has been widely interpreted as essentially an ideal of compassion, gentleness, humility, long-suffering, and magnanimous forgiveness of enemies. It is closely related to another aspect of Christian morals which we have already discussed— humanitarianism, or the feeling that all men are brothers. This conception of Christian character is very similar to the sort of ideal that grows up in a peaceful, industrial, democratic society.

This is enough to show the great complexity and variety of Christian conceptions of the ends and means of morality. The trend in modern times is certainly in the direction of a Christian conception of human happiness that is identical, as regards this world, with the secular, open-minded, experimental, democratic conception of human happiness which leaves it to each generation to decide what moral rules will be wisest and most likely to produce a good society everywhere throughout the earth. In so far as Christian morality means this sort of thing, discussion between Christians and others who want to see a happier world can proceed without difficulty, for such a discussion will be a factual one, drawing upon the best knowledge available in the natural and social sciences as well as upon everyday experience which cannot be expressed in exact scientific terms.

Liberal Judaism. The same thing may be said of Judaism as of Christianity. Orthodox Jewish morality includes many specific taboos regarding Sabbath observance, eating pork, and so on, and in so far as any violation of these taboos is regarded as an abomination to the Lord, or something intrinsically wrong, apart from its relation to human happiness, there is no room for rational discussion. But a liberal Jewish effort to discover the moral rules which will bring about most quickly a better social order would not be distinguishable from the morality of a liberal Christian or from a secular morality.

Those who regard morality as a means to the general end of human happiness and believe that wisdom in such matters is best attained through open-minded experimentation are in essential agreement, regardless of what religious label they go under.

Study Questions

1. What is the difference between a moral end and other ends (matters of taste)?
2. When one says that a "thing is right because it is right," is "right" an end in itself or a means to some other end?
3. How do persons who believe that certain duties are "right because they are right" resolve the mental conflict when one duty can be carried out only at the expense of another duty?
4. How do persons who believe that moral rules are means to some more general end resolve conflicts in duties?
5. What is the one tenet on which all Christians are agreed?
6. Does "love of one's neighbor" or "seeking the happiness of humanity" tell us all we need to know in order to set up a morality?
7. What are some of the meanings that "happiness" has?
8. State the method by which (a) conservative Protestants, (b) Catholics, and (c) liberal Christians determine God's will in regard to the meaning of true happiness and the means of attaining it.

9. Is there any difference in practice between liberal Protestants, liberal Jews, and other liberals?
10. What have been the moral taboos emphasized in the past by (a) conservative Protestants, (b) Catholics, and (c) orthodox Jews?
11. What are some of the virtues that make up the ideal of a Christian character?
12. Is any experimentalism to be found in any part of conservative Christian or Jewish morality?
13. Which ideals of life may be characterized as "sacrificial"?
14. What is the supreme end of Stoicism?
15. Name two well-known ancient Stoics.
16. Why is Stoicism unsatisfactory as an ideal of life? What is to be said in its favor?
17. What is the Heroic ideal of life?
18. What is the objection to making the strenuous life the supreme end?
19. Name the six ingredients of a happy life defined as the maximum satisfaction of basic desires.
20. Do Utilitarians regard virtues as ends in themselves or as means toward happiness?
21. What is the ideal of ethical individualism?

Questions for Thought and Discussion

1. In the *Republic* Plato presents this moral dilemma: A friend leaves a weapon with you and you promise to give it to him when he returns for it, but in the meantime he becomes insane and will probably kill you or others if you give him his weapon. Ought you to keep your promise and return his property to him? Or ought you to protect the life of yourself or others? On what principle would *you* resolve this moral conflict?
2. A deformed infant would be better off dead than alive. His existence casts a shadow over the life of his parents. If placed in an institution, he is a burden to the state. We could prevent this unhappiness by putting the infant to death, but on the other hand it is wrong to take a human life. What would you do (assuming

the laws of the state did not interfere)? On what principle would you base your decision?

3. You are a Protestant nurse. One of your Catholic patients in the hospital adheres to the regulation of refraining from eating meat on Friday. Do you feel any responsibility to provide this patient with a meat substitute on Fridays? If so, how do you reconcile this with your own practice of eating meat on Fridays?

   You are a Catholic taking care of a Protestant patient. Do you feel obliged to serve a meat substitute to the patient on Fridays? Or do you serve meat to the patient without any pangs of conscience? How do you account for your attitude?

4. Which ideal of life would you choose for yourself? Can you give any reason for adopting this ideal? Is this reason just a repetition of the ideal itself?

5. Which ideal of life is implied in Jesus' saying that "the Sabbath was made for man, not man for the Sabbath"?

6. Discuss dancing, card-playing, gambling, smoking, drinking, swearing, breaking the Sabbath, divorce, contraception, sterilization, abortion, euthanasia, and sun bathing in nudist colonies from the standpoint of human happiness defined as a well-rounded life on earth. Discuss them from the standpoint of eternal happiness in a future life.

7. If one says that "the end does not justify the means," does this imply that the avoidance of certain evil means is an end in itself? Do you think that some acts are intrinsically evil, i.e., eternally bad in themselves apart from their consequences?

8. Does happiness mean mere contentment or does your conception of it include adventure, risk, and living greatly?

9. Persons who are always seeking happiness never find it while those who are absorbed with various objects and enterprises and are not thinking about happiness often are the happiest people. (This is called "the hedonistic paradox." Hedonism is a Greek derivative meaning the pursuit of happiness or pleasure.) Does

this prove that one ought not to set up happiness as the supreme end? If not, what does it indicate? What do these words of Jesus mean: "He that findeth his life shall lose it and he that loseth his life shall find it"?

10. If a utopian society should be achieved in which there were no more serious political, economic, or social problems and no great suffering or maladjustment, this might destroy the stimulus for great literature. Do you think it would?

If so, would you rather live in an unhappy society which could produce great literature or in a happy society with mediocre literature?

11. Which ideal of happiness is implied in the democratic doctrine of "life, liberty, and the pursuit of happiness"?

12. John Stuart Mill said that he would rather be a human being dissatisfied than a pig satisfied. How about you?

13. The Bible says "he that increaseth knowledge increaseth sorrow." Also you have heard that "ignorance is bliss." Would you rather have an education and be unhappy or be ignorant and happy?

14. How is your life at present (or your plans for the future) related to satisfying the six basic needs of health, social status, intimate affection, recreation, parental feeling, and rightness? Are you making a realistic approach to your problems or are you employing "escape mechanisms" to avoid coming to grips with some problems? Are any of your present adjustments likely to contribute to failure in the end?

Books to Read

The Bible, The Gospel of Matthew.

Castell, Alburey: *An Introduction to Modern Philosophy*. New York. Macmillan. 1943. Section on Nietzsche.

Durant, Will: *The Story of Philosophy*, new ed. rev. Garden City Publishing Company. 1938. Chapters on Spinoza and Nietzsche.

Epictetus: *The Discourses of Epictetus: with the Encheiridion and Fragments*. Everyman's Library, Bohn's Classical Library. 1906.

Hyde, William DeWitt: *The Five Great Philosophies of Life.* New York. Macmillan. 1924.

Mill, John Stuart: *Autobiography.* New York. Columbia University Press. 1924.

Pressey, Sidney L., Janney, Joseph Elliott, and Kuhlen, Raymond G: *Life—A Psychological Survey.* New York and London. Harper. 1939. Chapter VII.

XI

The Greatest-Happiness Principle

THE PRECEDING chapter has presented five ideals of life. The present will deal with some of the problems arising in the application of these ideals. After an ideal, or supreme end of life, has been adopted, the main problem for a morality is to *maximize* this ideal—throughout the life of a given individual and throughout society in the lives of as many human beings as possible. Now we cannot get very far in discussing the problem of maximizing ideals *in general*, but in order to say anything significant or work out principles of practical value we must have a particular ideal in mind which we wish to realize. That means that before we can proceed farther we must select for further development one of the philosophies of life which we have been discussing.

The ideal that we shall develop throughout the remainder of this book may be considered any one of the last three, depending upon the point of view. As between the third and fourth ideals —the maximum satisfaction of basic needs and the maximum freedom—the difference is largely academic. If we were to ask how we should go about achieving either of these goals in society, the answer would probably be the same in each case. That is to say, if we wanted to encourage the broadest, richest type of happiness, we would do it by giving people a liberal education, providing the best opportunities for earning a comfortable living, and then leaving them as free as possible to work out their own salvation. But this is precisely what the advocate of ethical individualism would do. We have also seen how the abundant life which the liberal Christian seeks for all humanity is in practice the same as the well-rounded happiness which the Utilitarian philosopher may describe in more academic terms. Hence, while in a textbook the terminology which we shall use will be necessarily chiefly academic, the principles of conduct developed will in no essential differ from those which are being expressed in religious terms by liberal men and women throughout the modern world.

The essential element in these liberal approaches to ethics is the tendency to keep the formula for happiness general enough so as not to commit us to any fixed and unchangeable rules of conduct. Moral rules must be kept in the category of means, not ends. That is to say, they must be kept flexible. Indeed, even the end—human happiness—is flexible in that it is general enough to include all possible demands of future generations.

Experimentalism vs. Fixation

In later chapters we shall find that the difference between this conception of happiness and that represented by other points of view can be summarized best by the phrase: *experimentalism versus fixation.* It matters little about any academic quibbles over the meaning of happiness as long as all parties to the argument are willing to leave it to each generation to work out its own conception of happiness and decide what means are best suited to its ends, in view of the circumstances existing at that time. Moral experimentalism means that we do not regard any rule of conduct as eternally and intrinsically right. Rather our morality will always be subject to criticism and revision on the basis of its serving or not serving the end of human happiness. And each case is to be judged on its own merits.

> "New occasions make new duties;
> Time makes ancient good uncouth.
> They must upward still and onward
> Who would keep abreast of Truth."

The philosophical term "Utilitarianism" originated as a description of this experimental attitude toward moral rules. The rightness of any act, Utilitarian philosophers said, is determined by its *utility* in producing human happiness. "Utility" here, however, means usefulness in the broadest sense of the word. Utilitarianism does not mean that an act is moral if it is useful in a narrow, practical, immediate, or selfish way. It means that *an act is moral if it is useful for producing the greatest happiness in the long run and in a social sense.*

Once morality is placed in the category of *means* to the general end of human happiness, the Utilitarian's problem is simply to trace the *consequences* of various acts to see whether they produce the greatest possible happiness or not. Moral problems thus become factual problems and their solution depends upon the amount of science and common sense that we can bring to bear upon them.

How Is Each Act to be Judged?

Direct Consequences and By-Products. In calculating consequences it is important to have an eye to the *by-products* of our actions as well as to the *direct consequences.* For example, when we tell a lie there is not merely the immediate result which we aim to achieve but there is an effect upon our character and the character and attitudes of others. Telling one lie makes it easier to tell the next one, and if we are not careful we will develop the habit of taking the easy way out in every case instead of facing the music and telling the plain truth. Likewise, our conduct may influence others so that the habit of lying spreads. And lastly confidence may be undermined. The one who lies expects the same thing in others so that he is suspicious of them, and of course, they are suspicious of him.

This pictures the by-products of lying at their worst. In cases in which a person lies from altruistic motives, however, there is less likelihood of general distrust being created. Also the individual who lies for the good of others is not so likely to develop the habit as a personal weakness, though even in altruistic lying there is no doubt some cultivation of an inclination to use deception. It is easy to become so habituated to being diplomatic and tactful that we lose our capacity to deal with situations in a forthright fashion. Nevertheless, most of us feel that under some circumstances the bad effects of lying are negligible and so we approve of "white lies," as we call them. We agree with Aristotle in calling it the vice of "tactlessness" to tell the truth, the whole truth, and nothing but the truth at all times. We spare people much unhappiness by observing certain social amenities, such as not telling a woman how terrible a new hat looks, or by replying to the question "How are you?" with a "Very well, thank you!", although we may feel anything but well. And we take this sort of deception so much for granted that it remains well compartmentalized and does not undermine our capacity to be truthful in more important matters. Similarly, lying in order to save lives is certainly so easily distinguished from the lying of a weak character that there would be little danger here of transfer of habit.*

Of course, there is no denying that there are difficult, borderline cases that are not so easily disposed of, and a great deal of wisdom and caution is needed in reasoning through them. The main point we wish to make, however, is that a morality based upon calculation of consequences will be shortsighted and sometimes dangerous, unless *both* the by-products and direct results of our conduct are taken into account. This places upon the individual a heavy responsibility and demands the exercise of all the intelligence and experience that he has at his command.

The person who says "I cannot tell a lie" saves himself the trouble of thinking. He will still need some intelligence and experience in applying his morality, but he is spared much responsibility. He misses a freedom, however. It is so with all the exigencies of life and the rules that older moralities have devised to meet them.

Particular and General Consequences. Several of the chapters which are to follow will contain illustrations drawn from the medical and nursing professions which will make clearer the difference between Utilitarian morality, which judges each act by its particular consequences, and other moralities which regard certain acts as intrinsically evil. Christian morality in so far as it is of this latter type is based upon St. Paul's injunction that we should never do evil "that good may come of it." This implies a fixed and unchangeable list of evil acts. On the other hand, in Utilitarian morality and in some liberal forms of Christianity and Judaism, what is meant by an evil act is not one which is *always* wrong but one which *generally* results in unhappiness. Hence, the question "Ought we to do evil that

---

* Example: Concealing a piece of news from a patient whose life might be endangered by hearing the truth; or giving a fictitious reason to a theater audience for leaving the building, in order to save them from a fire of which they were not yet aware.

good may come of it?" means "Ought we to do that which usually results in unhappiness but in this particular case will result in more happiness than unhappiness?" When we conclude that we ought to do evil, this sounds paradoxical or contradictory. But it is not, for in a morality based upon consequences, an act may be called good or evil from the standpoint of (1) its *usual* consequences and (2) its consequences in the *particular* case. An act which is evil in general may be good in particular and we ought therefore to do it, for it is the particular consequences of an act that determines whether we ought to do it or not. Lying, for example, is bad in general but is justifiable if employed to foil a criminal, to prevent an insane person from doing harm, to prevent capture by an enemy in war, to maintain the amenities of life, etc. Taking human life is bad in general but it may be justified in self-defense, the enforcement of international peace, the prevention of crime, euthanasia, and therapeutic abortions. Differences of opinion regarding these illustrations would represent different calculations of consequences.

In most cases, of course, the general tendency of an act coincides with its particular tendency so that there is no conflict. And, as a matter of fact, we take this so much for granted that we usually depend upon general rules without bothering to calculate the consequences of each act. In such situations all ethical philosophies follow parallel lines. Only when a particular case is strikingly different from the general rule does one feel the need of ethical reflection by which he can judge the act on its own merits. *Whether an act should be judged on the basis of its particular consequences or not* is the crucial element that divides moralities into two great conflicting classes. It will be this factor more than any other that will determine our choices in the chapters which follow.

Whose Happiness Ought We to Seek?

We have been talking about calculating the consequences of our acts in terms of happiness but we have not grappled with the question: *whose* happiness are we to be concerned about? That may seem a foolish question to a nurse, who by her very choice of a profession shows that she is interested in others as well as herself. Even so, there still remains the problem of deciding how much weight one should give to self-interest, interest in family and friends, and interest in humanity at large. To what extent should we sacrifice our own interest for that of our family, or vice versa? To what extent should we risk the welfare of ourselves or our families for the sake of humanity?

There is also a theoretical question that has long interested philosophers. That is, assuming that one has both selfish and altruistic interests, is it possible to derive all one's altruistic conduct from enlightened self-interest? If one is really wise in trying to get the most happiness for himself, will he necessarily conclude that the best way to be sure of his own happiness is to be considerate of others? In other words, does it always pay to be good? On the other hand, suppose we dislike the idea of basing our morality on self-interest and would rather base it upon a kindly interest in the welfare of human beings everywhere. Could we derive all our conduct from this principle of the greatest happiness for all humanity? Could we show that even the things we do for ourselves are just designed to keep us fit for the task of serving humanity? Would this be a realistic morality?

Enlightened Self-Interest. Let us consider first whether a morality could be based upon enlightened self-interest. There is no doubt that a good deal of our moral training is based upon this assumption that it is advantageous to be good. We tell children that if they are mean and selfish with others, nobody will like them. And later we impress them with the fact that throughout life, in business or in personal affairs, honesty is the best policy. "Crime does not pay."

To a great extent this is true. And in a well-ordered society it would be very true that an anti-social person would be looked down upon and would find it much more advantageous to be good rather than bad. Unfortunately, in an imperfect society there are groups that work at cross purposes with one another, and some persons who are a menace to the whole society may be honored in their own neighborhood or gang. Also, persons who are disloyal to larger social interests may obtain influential positions in politics or in police departments and may connive with criminals in evading punishment. So it is possible for a criminal to grow wealthy and powerful and enjoy prestige among his fellow gangsters and even live to a ripe old age. Of course, many or perhaps most criminals come to grief, but it is impossible to prove that this is necessarily the case. Furthermore in matters that do not involve a violation of the law, we often see people get ahead in business or in professions by methods that are none too honorable. So the proposition that the good always prosper and the wicked perish has never been demonstrated to the satisfaction of those who are wise to the ways of the world. The attempt to base morality upon rational self-interest has been, at least in part, a failure ever since Job cried out against the injustice of the world and asked, "Wherefore do the wicked live, become old, yea, are mighty in power?"

There is another reason, too, why morality cannot, or should not, be based entirely upon the doctrine of enlightened self-interest. Would we enjoy living with people whose only reason for treating their fellows considerately was that it *paid?* No. We like to have as friends persons who are spontaneously and often selflessly kind and generous. We feel much more secure with them than with someone who treats us well only because he calculates he will gain thereby. We are afraid that some time his calculations may not work out right. Unselfishness by the route of selfishness is almost a contradiction in terms, for it is not likely that enlightened selfishness alone would produce a society of unselfish, agreeable companions.

At the same time, in a world in which right triumphs with difficulty we have to snatch at whatever help we can find. Therefore, in so far as we can convince selfish people that it will be to their interest to help others, so much the better. Such an appeal has sometimes been made to wealthy people who have been told that, if they allowed poverty and disease to exist in the slums, they themselves would fall victim to some of the germs which do not know that they are supposed to stay on the other side of the tracks. Or, in depressions the argument is used that if we don't provide adequate relief or employment, the discontented masses will riot and turn things upside down. While it is deplorable that there are people who can be moved only by such arguments, still it is better that they be moved by this appeal to selfishness than not be moved at all.

On the international scene, where morality exists at a lower level than in local communities, enlightened selfishness would go a long way toward eliminating war and raising the standard of living of all nations. An example is what the views of economists could accomplish if generally understood and accepted. Thus, we would be better off in the long run by lowering tariff barriers and opening up the channels of trade to all nations. But the appeal to self-interest here is less objectionable, partly because we are used to it in economic matters and partly because selfish cooperation of nations would certainly be better than the selfish throat-cutting we have known in the past.

Interest in Humanity. At the opposite pole from the attempt to base morality upon rational self-interest is the belief that all conduct can be subordinated to the principle of the greatest happiness of the greatest number. This is a much more palatable doctrine, though probably no more true to reality, than enlightened self-interest. Progress might be greatly accelerated if everybody could forget himself and his family and think primarily of humanity. But it is doubtful whether we would enjoy the company of people who could sacrifice their intimate, personal interests to such an abstract ideal. The following story will illustrate this.

A famous scientist is hiking in the Alps with his wife, for whom he cares a great deal. They are tied together with a rope to aid one another in difficult feats of climbing. It is very important that the scientist should not lose his life, as he has just about finished some experiments which will be of tremendous importance to millions of human beings. Let us say that he is on the verge of discovering some new source of energy which will replace our diminishing supplies of coal and oil. But he has come to the Alps for a little relaxation just before completing his great work. Imagine, then, the moral dilemma which he faces when suddenly his wife slips and falls over a ledge. He struggles to pull her back with the rope by which they are tied together but his strength gives out and slowly she drags him down to meet the same death as herself in the abyss below. What should he do? The happiness of millions dictates that he should take out his knife and cut the rope, so as to save himself for the completion of his scientific work. But could he do it?

Could he look down into his wife's pleading eyes and yet proceed to cut the rope and let her plunge down to her doom alone? Certainly he could not do this, no matter what the future of mankind, nor would we expect him to do so.

Plurality of Interests. This shows that it is too much to expect human beings to sacrifice close personal ties for a remote, abstract interest in humanity. Indeed, considering how little concern for humanity actually exists, we should be thankful if a person devotes even a moderate amount of his time and energy to such a broad interest, without demanding that he make it his supreme end. A more practicable ideal would be that of expecting each person to have a reasonable amount of concern about all the people with whom he is associated, both near and far, as well as considerable interest in his own well-being. In other words, the moral ideal would consist of a *plurality of interests*—self interest, primary-group interests (interest in family, friends, neighbors, or fellow-workers), and secondary-group interests (interests ranging from the local community to all living humanity and posterity).

This would be more in accord with the actual attitude of good people. They do not have a hierarchy of interests, all neatly subordinated to some one supreme end, but their interests are coordinate, that is, they exist side by side, with varying degrees of intensity. Usually the strongest interest centers about self or family or very intimate friends, and other interests grow progressively weaker as we get farther away from home. This leaves us, however, with the problem of determining what is the ideal strength for each of these interests.

Harmony of Interests. How much is a reasonable or legitimate interest in self, primary group, or secondary group? What constitutes a well-balanced life in this respect? It would be convenient if a precise formula could be given so that we might know on every occasion whether we are too selfish, too family-minded, or even too much preoccupied with remote interests. But nothing more than a general suggestion can be offered. In actual life each one has to depend upon his own, often vague, experience, which of course changes as the needs and experience of society change.

Those of us who are already concerned to a considerable

extent about humanity throughout the earth would like to see everyone possess enough of the broader type of interest to bring about a world society in which there will no longer be a conflict between various group interests. And anyone who has ever suffered from a mental conflict occasioned by the necessity of sacrificing one interest for another would like to live in a world in which there would be a harmony of all interests with no one called upon to sacrifice legitimate interests. Hence there arises a supplementary moral end or objective, namely *harmony*, which has the function of regulating our primary interests in self, small-groups, and large-groups. *The ideal weight, therefore, which should be given to each of these interests is that which the members of a perfectly harmonious world-society would give them. That is what we mean when we say that a certain amount of interest in self, family, and humanity in general, is reasonable or legitimate.* It is the degree of interest that would not cause the sacrifice of other harmonizable interests in a well-ordered society.

Conflict of Interests. In an imperfect world, however, we are sometimes forced to choose between two entirely legitimate interests. For example, a newspaper writer may have to choose between suppressing facts which he thinks people ought to know and losing his job. The loss of a job, particularly during a depression, may mean the ruin of his family. He is thus forced to choose between his concern for the larger social welfare and the welfare of his family. Teachers sometimes have to make similar choices. In industrial strife, too, workers sometimes are called upon to inflict hardships upon their families for the sake of their trade union principles. In professions, such as medicine and nursing, difficult decisions involving public and private interests have to be made at times. And in war almost anyone may be called upon to sacrifice interests of self and family for the good of nation and humanity.

In all these cases morality does not give any clear direction, except in a great crisis, such as war, where all are agreed that sacrifices of self and family are in order. In bitter industrial warfare, too, much is demanded of workers by their fellows. But in most other cases the tendency is for us not to demand the sacrifice of family or self for a larger ideal. In history and

literature we may romanticize about the nobility of such sacrifices but in everyday life, under ordinary circumstances, we
usually call people foolish for making martyrs of themselves.
We are not too hard on others in our moral judgments and we
do not exact too much of them for the reason that we would
not like to have too much demanded of ourselves. So in general
we adopt the policy of encouraging people to compromise and
salvage as much of both public and private interests as they
can. Thus we hope to muddle through to a better day when
choices between legitimate interests will no longer be forced
upon us and we shall no longer have to say with Hamlet:

> The time is out of joint. O cursed spite,
> That ever I was born to set it right!

The Means to Happiness

Having set up our moral end, we ought logically to consider
next the means which will best achieve it for us. These means
may be divided into two large classes consisting of (1) the
general rules of morality, especially those applying to personal
conduct, and (2) the social, political, and economic institutions
under which we live. Both of these will be discussed throughout
the remainder of this book. Here we may simply remark that
most of us feel quite certain that the democratic principles of
liberty and equality provide the best means for achieving the
greatest happiness of humanity. Democracy, however, in order
to be a really effective instrument for human welfare needs to
be more than a mere slogan. It will require some hard thinking
and hard work to make it mean all that it can mean in our lives.

The Trend Toward Cultural Unity

A final word should be said about the problem of moral
agreement. If each person works out his own morality, limited
only by the definition that morality consists of those desires
which we expect others to support us in, what guarantee do we
have that people will get together on the same program of
social improvement? Some persons may fear that only anarchy
would result from such a conception of morality. How can the
thought-out conclusions of individual happiness-seekers result
in anything like a social order? This fear neglects the fact that

human nature and experience in society are uniform enough to insure a great deal of agreement at any time and ultimately practically universal agreement. The fact that morality in any system consists of desires which we desire others to share provides the social interaction or give-and-take which is needed to iron out differences and produce a common culture. Also there is something in the very nature of the broad humanitarianism of the ideal of a well-rounded life which makes it particularly adaptable and on this account likely to achieve a permanent stability. All narrower nationalistic or tribalistic enthusiasms in a world of expanding social contacts are bound to produce friction and war, bringing unhappiness to victor and vanquished alike. Only a universal morality which takes into account the legitimate interests of all peoples can survive, once it has been established. It is like truth, or science, in this respect. Superstition and error of any sort have within themselves seeds of their own destruction, i.e., an incompatible element that will always cause mental discontent in some quarter until it is finally replaced by a truth which will permanently harmonize with all experience. The guarantee of cultural unity throughout the world is that there is only one science and one morality that can stand the test of time. Only that which takes into account all humanity and all experience can survive.

Study Questions

1. What is the meaning of moral experimentalism or utilitarianism? Does utilitarianism mean judging conduct by its utility in a narrow, practical sense?
2. What two kinds of consequences ought we to take into account in judging an act?
3. Show why some lies are considered "white lies" and others not.
4. What would St. Paul say to the principle that the end justifies the means?
5. How do you explain the paradox that it is right to do wrong under certain circumstances?
6. Is it true that goodness invariably leads to happiness, and wickedness to unhappiness? To what extent are goodness and happiness correlated?

7. Would social life based solely upon enlightened self-interest be agreeable?
8. How would enlightened self-interest prevent war?
9. Can a good person's life *really* be organized entirely about the principle of the greatest happiness of the greatest number? Is the illustration of the scientist and his wife sound evidence for this?
10. Describe a morality based upon a plurality of coordinate interests or loyalties.
11. How can we determine what is a reasonable or legitimate interest in self, family, or society at large?
12. When legitimate interests conflict in our present society, what attitude do people usually take toward sacrificing family or self for the general welfare?
13. What is the relation of democracy to utilitarian morality?
14. If everyone works out his own morality, what guarantee is there that social agreement will ever be attained? What is the only morality that does not carry with it the seeds of its own destruction?

Questions for Thought and Discussion

1. An experimental or utilitarian morality advocates keeping all rules flexible. Is there any element of fixity in such a system? Compare with George Bernard Shaw's maxim: The golden rule is that there is no golden rule. Is the open-minded person open-minded about open-mindedness? Is the tolerant person tolerant of intolerance? Apparently every system of thought or morals or politics in the last analysis contains some fixed, dogmatic principle. When is fixity or dogmatism justifiable and when not?
2. Jesus said that "the Sabbath was made for man, not man for the Sabbath." St. Paul said that we should not do evil "that good may come of it." Which of these represents the utilitarian attitude toward moral rules and which implies that certain acts are intrinsically wrong regardless of the consequences. With which do you agree?
3. "We become the things we do" is an argument against

using evil means for good ends. To what extent is it valid?

4. A young woman lost her husband in an automobile accident soon after marriage. For many weeks afterwards she kept saying, "I must have committed some very great sin to have deserved this." What belief regarding the correlation of virtue and happiness did she apparently have?

5. Is there any sense in which a' good person is necessarily happy? What is the meaning of: "Virtue is its own reward"? What did Plato mean when he said that "no evil can come to a good man either in life or after death"? Does he refer to evil in the inner or external sense of the word?

6. If a friend of yours had a revolver and you knew that she planned to commit suicide, would it be right for you to steal her revolver to prevent this?

7. If you were guiding a party through a desert and lost your way and after several days it became evident that there was just enough food to enable you and one other member of the party to get back to an oasis, whom would you select to go with you? One of the party is a gentle old lady. Another is an eminent scientist who has just made a discovery that will solve the problem of heat and power for billions of human beings after our coal and oil supplies have been exhausted, but he has not published his results yet. A third member of the party is the person to whom you are engaged to be married.

8. Suppose that a miser has a large amount of money stored in a vault. He has kept no record of the amount, no one is aware that he has accumulated a fortune, and he leaves no will. You have nursed him in his declining years and are the only one who shares his secret. When the miser dies, you have a choice, let us say, between (a) notifying the public authorities so that the Probate Court may distribute the money among undeserving and spendthrift relatives, and (b) turning the money over to various poor families who need it

badly or perhaps to some hospital that needs funds. Which would you do? Opponents of utilitarianism have argued that since no one knows about the existence of this money, there would be no bad by-products in the way of encouragement to others to steal or take the law into their own hands, and therefore utilitarian reasoning would lead us to conclude that it is right to steal the money, since the greatest happiness of the greatest number would result. Yet common-sense tells us that it would be wrong. This proves, they say, that we cannot always judge behavior by its consequences. Are these critics of utilitarianism right? Have they taken into account *all* the by-products?

9. We believe that in a democracy we are inclined to have regard for the happiness of all humanity. Yet we refuse to give emigrants from poor countries a chance to improve their fortunes by coming to America, for we say that the admission of millions of immigrants would overpopulate our country and lower our standards of living. Is this evidence that it is unrealistic to try to base morality upon an interest in humanity at large? Is there any way of showing that this apparently selfish and nationalistic policy will really work to the advantage of the whole earth in the long run?

10. If it is true that there is a trend toward a common morality throughout the earth and if this universal morality turns out to be utilitarian, will this uniformity produce cultural stagnation? In other words, is more progress made when there are a number of clashing ideals in the world? Science has become international. Has this resulted in stagnation? Is utilitarianism analogous to science?

Books to Read

Mill, John Stuart: *Utilitarianism*. Everyman's Library. 1926.
Russell, Bertrand: *The Conquest of Happiness*. Garden City Publishing Co. 1933.

XII

Moral Conflicts in Medicine and Nursing

P·ROFESSIONAL CODES. In every occupation or profession there are dozens of rules or customs which past experience has proved to be of value in promoting the welfare of (a) those engaged in the occupation, (b) those being immediately served, or (c) the general public. Some of these rules are explicit and may be published in a code adopted by an organization, while some of them may remain always in the form of a loosely defined, general understanding. The American Medical Association, for example, has written a code for physicians, but nurses have never "frozen" their moral rules into a code subscribed to by all nursing organizations.

The nursing profession has been wise in so doing, for thus its ethics is likely to be more responsive to new conditions, or, in other words, more adaptable. A written code usually includes concessions to dogmatic, well organized, highly vocal minorities, and the more liberal members of the nursing profession ought to keep clear of such commitments. Once a code is adopted, it is very difficult to get it changed, because of inertia if nothing else.

Individual Interpretations. Whether, however, a code is written or is just a matter of custom, the really difficult problems arise in interpreting it and in deciding whether circumstances justify violating any of its rules. When we open up the question of interpreting or breaking a rule, a welter of conflicting claims crowd in upon us—the interests of self, profession, patient and society. How to decide these claims? It would be fine if we could state a scientific, mathematical formula for resolving all conflicts, but unfortunately that is not possible. Moral decisions have to be based in the final analysis upon the rather vague and subjective experience of the individual. Each individual has a little different feeling as to where to draw the line and each feels the tug of loyalties within him in somewhat different proportions. Fortunately, however, we all have similar natures and have been reared in about the same social environment and with approximately the same education, and the results of our moral calculations, therefore, exhibit a good deal of uniformity in spite of being based upon feelings whose strength cannot be measured.

For example, even though there is no mathematical formula to guide people in deciding when it is all right to break the rule of truthfulness and tell a white lie, nevertheless there is large agreement among us as to the circumstances that justify this. Our sense about the desirability of making an exception almost amounts to another rule, as may be seen in our having a common word "white" to designate such lawful exceptions. At the same time, while we are thus pretty safe in most cases in allowing the individual to use his discretion about telling white lies, some individuals, who are unusually callous or selfish or cowardly or weak, will take advantage of the privilege of making exceptions and will lie when there is no social justification for it. Thus, with individualism and intelligence in modern morality there goes some risk of abuse, but we believe that the risk is worth taking in view of the opportunity for more rapid moral progress afforded by a flexible morality.

About all the moralist can do is to say to each one: Think about all the factors that enter into the situation and then make the best decision you can. But what are the factors in a situation which we ought to take into account in order that our judgment will have a moral quality and not represent mere caprice or wilfulness? First of all, as we have seen in a previous chapter, we must form the habit of thinking in terms of the *consequences* of our behavior. But we must think not merely of the *direct consequences* but of the *by-products*, or the general, or more distant future effects of our conduct. Calculation of the by-products will usually emphasize the interests of society at large and the maintenance of the sort of character in the individual which is advantageous to society, while our thought about direct consequences usually refers to particular individuals who will be benefited. Thus when a white lie is told, the immediate effect is to benefit some person, e.g., a patient who seems unreasonable, a patient whose life may be endangered by the shock of a true piece of news, or a crowd in a theater whose lives may be saved from a stampede by a concealment of the fact that there is a fire in the building. On the other hand, there is the possibility that the habit of taking the easy way out and lying may be strengthened in us by this act. Also a patient whom we have deceived may find this out and henceforth have less confidence in doctors, nurses, and hospitals in general. It is especially dangerous to try to manage children by lying to them, for they are very keen at detecting falsehoods and, not understanding adult discriminations regarding white lies, they may form the habit of being suspicious and of being deceitful themselves. Obviously, therefore, the emergency must be very great in order for us to be sure that the good consequences of a lie more than counterbalance its bad general tendencies. Unless the evil effects of the truth are so obvious and serious that they strike us with great force and unless there is no other way out, we should not even entertain the question of whether to tell the truth or not. When at all in doubt about whether a lie is a "white" one, it is a good policy to decide in favor of the truth.

These are the sort of considerations that enter into those occasional cases in which we may be justified in debating the advisability of making an exception to a good rule. For the most part, however, rules represent the greatest happiness of all concerned and they contain so much of the accumulated wisdom of humanity or of a given profession that it is both unnecessary and unwise to tamper with them. They should become a second nature with us, violated only in those rare instances when their ineptness strikes us in the face, so to speak.

But we have set for ourselves in this chapter the problem of dealing with moral conflicts which call for an exception to some part of a professional code or to some general rule of morality. Let us, therefore, first enumerate some of the time-honored rules of medicine and nursing and then consider difficulties which may arise if these rules are adhered to too rigidly.

Some Good Rules

Here are some rules which we may recognize as contributing to the welfare of nurses, doctors, patients, and the general public:

1. Always do what is best for the patient.
2. Avoid criticism of doctors or nurses in the presence of patients or other laymen.
3. Carry out the doctor's orders.
4. Tell the truth.
5. Regard confidences as sacred.
6. Avoid intimacy with patients.
7. Avoid discussing religion or politics with patients.
8. Refrain from accepting gifts from patients.
9. Avoid doing anything for which you might be sued.
10. Refrain from countenancing commercialism in the medical or nursing profession.
11. Discourage self-medication in patients.

Can Good Rules Go Wrong?

(1) Our first rule, *always do what is best for the patient,* certainly sounds like a rule that would always hold good. But we shall see in the course of our discussion of other rules that even this supremely important principle may sometimes be in conflict with some other rule of ethics and something has to be sacrificed somewhere. Just what and how much is to be sacrificed when duties conflict is a decision that a nurse has to become used to making.

Sometimes it is possible to reconcile a sacrifice of the interest of particular patients with the interests of the general public. For example, a public health nurse may be employed in a community in which there is inadequate medical care and she may see enough work to occupy her time twenty-four hours of the day. She may devote herself heroically to this task at the sacrifice of her own time and at the risk of her health. But there is a limit beyond which she should not go. The welfare of the community itself may be endangered, if she so continually deprives herself of rest and relaxation that she finally breaks down under the strain. Furthermore, it is a sad fact but a true one that sometimes the government and other public agencies cannot be stirred into action as long as some devoted worker is willing to make personal sacrifices to keep a service from breaking down. Thus, the ultimate good of the public may be served by sacrificing the good of particular patients, however heart-rending this may be. And, of course, while a nurse is expected to be generous and selfless up to a certain point, she too as an individual has rights. But just how far the welfare of the patient is allowed to encroach upon the ultimate rights of the nurse or the ultimate welfare of the community is something which the nurse must decide on the basis of her own experience.

Incidentally, in an ideal society no such forced choices between duties to patient, self, and community would have to be made. In fact, an ideal society may be defined as just that kind of society in which there is a harmony of interests instead of a conflict of legitimate loyalties. We ought accordingly not to expend all of our energy on struggling with the hopeless dilemmas of an imperfect society but we should devote some of our thought to reconstructing the whole society politically and economically so that eventually we shall not so often be confronted with moral and professional dilemmas.

(2) In *the rule against criticizing a colleague* the medical profession has developed a means of protecting itself against (a) an ignorant public and (b) unscrupulous physicians. A well educated person might be able to hear a frank criticism of a physician and still have confidence in medical science in general, but those who do not have enough education to understand the sound foundations of medicine have to depend upon the prestige and solidarity of the medical profession in order to have the confidence in it that is required for best results. The rule of putting up a united front, therefore, really serves the patient as much as the physician. And the same is true as regards physicians who would compete unfairly by running down their more competent colleagues, if they had a chance. The code not only protects physicians but also patients against such unscrupulous persons. Even where there is no intention of damaging the reputation of a colleague, all of us are prone to engage in a good deal of loose talk and a blunt rule against any criticism

whatsoever of our fellow-workers is an effective check upon such thoughtless gossip. This is true of all professions.

But what if a physician really is incompetent and ought to be criticized? Or what if he is being sued for malpractice? Ought a colleague to testify against him? The lay public feels that it is outrageous for a physician not to testify against one of his fellows when he knows that he has been negligent or has taken a case though unfit to handle it. Yet the matter is not as simple as it seems. In the first place, in every community there are some persons who are ready to sue for malpractice on the slightest pretext, especially when egged on by a dishonest lawyer. Even the best physicians may be victimized by such people, and if physicians were in the habit of testifying frequently against one another this would lend encouragement to crooks everywhere and there would be many more suits than there are. Besides, it is not easy to prove malpractice in a single case and so physicians would normally be wary anyhow of asserting negligence or incompetence except in the most flagrant cases.

Nurses are confronted by similar problems of professional behavior. Originally, when nurses were regarded as little better than the servants of physicians, the moral decisions which the former had to make were not as complex as they are today. The nurse was not permitted to criticize the physician because she was relatively uninformed and was not supposed to understand the methods which he was employing but merely to carry them out blindly. Now, with the greatly improved scientific background which nurses receive as part of their study, they can recognize medical incompetence pretty well and they feel tempted at times to report it. Also, since a nurse can herself be sued for carrying out a doctor's orders when they are obviously wrong, she has a much heavier responsibility than ever before. The duty of nurses today, therefore, in regard to criticizing doctors is twofold: While working with a physician and carrying out his prescriptions it would not be fair to him nor good for the patient to undermine confidence in his medical competence. And also the same reasons given above for doctors' "sticking together" apply to nurses in their relation to physicians and in their relation to other nurses. But, just as among physicians there are flagrant cases which justify breaking the rule of non-criticism, so do such cases sometimes occur in a nurse's experience.

Loyalty to superior, loyalty to profession, loyalty to patient, and loyalty to community—all these are *usually* served by the professional code. But in the occasional instance where some loyalties are served by a rule and some are not, the conflict may be so striking that the question of making an exception cannot be put aside. Then the nurse must weigh the opposing claims against one another, make her decision, and hope that it works out for the best. She must realize that she is playing with dynamite, and it is usually our duty *not* to play with dynamite, but on the other hand sometimes it *is* our duty to take this risk.

Better than having to resolve such conflicts individually would be to work under a system which contained orderly processes for preventing or controlling incompetence. We have been moving rapidly toward such a goal in the past generation. Now there are scarcely any third-rate medical schools (i.e., schools operated on an irresponsible, commercial basis) and there are only a few surviving schools that fall short of the Class A rating of the American Medical Association. This means that henceforth we can be pretty sure that any physician who has survived the ordeal of regular medical training is reasonably competent and in most cases honest. In addition to this, methods of recognizing and licensing specialists are improving. And, finally, as medicine becomes more institutionalized and all surgeons come under the supervision and discipline of well-organized medical staffs in large hospitals, incompetence can be dealt with quietly and effectively within the medical profession without the public's becoming aware of any disunity. The same thing, of course, has long been true of nurses engaged in public health and institutional nursing.

(3) Just as a good rule can go wrong if a physician or nurse is *never* willing to expose the incompetence of a colleague or superior, so also can the rule of always *obeying the doctor's orders* sometimes lead to fatal consequences if adhered to without exception. Obviously it would be an affront to a physician to have his orders constantly reviewed, criticized, or nullified by a nurse who had had little training of the sort required in pre-

scribing medicines. But sometimes even the best of physicians may absent-mindedly make a mistake, and in such cases he should be thankful that a nurse calls an error to his attention rather than stand on his dignity and assume an air of infallibility, frightening away any intelligent assistance a nurse may give him. A really great physician will not resent some questioning of his orders, if done in the right spirit, even though occasionally it may prove unwarranted. He and his profession have enough reserves of honor and prestige without having to struggle for it over little things. It is the physician who is insecure personally who demands slavish obedience from nurses.

The nurse must be prepared, however, to face the unjust wrath of such small-minded physicians when necessary. If she feels certain that a serious error has been made, her duty to her patient requires that she run the risk of an explosion from the doctor when she communicates with him. This danger can be reduced somewhat, even with the most irascible of physicians, if a tactful and respectful approach is made. Well chosen words, which subtly salve the ego of those who yearn for deference, may spell the difference between good and bad feelings between physician and nurse. It is unfortunate and unjust that some adults—sometimes very distinguished ones—have to be humored and handled with gloves on. Yet it is one of the hard realities of professional life that such persons exist, and we have to deal with them accordingly.

Once in a great while the nurse may encounter an even more difficult problem than questioning a physician about an order. Sometimes it is impossible to get in touch with the physician, and there may be no intern or superior in the nursing staff available. So the nurse may have to take it upon herself to modify the physician's order, if she feels an overpowering certainty that he has made a mistake or a condition has arisen which he did not foresee. Such a contingency is very unlikely to arise in a large institution but in private nursing it may sometimes happen that it is impossible to find another physician to consult in the absence of one's own. The nurse simply has to accept the fact that at such times her position is one of the most difficult in the world—responsibility without authority.

A final question may be raised regarding the morality of

cooperating with a physician in case one believes that he is doing something unethical, or even illegal. For example, what should a nurse do if she finds herself on a case involving a therapeutic abortion but she is a strict adherent of a religion that does not regard this as moral? It is generally agreed that if she discovers this when she is in the midst of a case and it is impossible to have another nurse replace her, it is her duty to remain because the life of the patient may depend upon her. On the other hand, if she knows in advance what kind of operation is to be performed, her religious scruples may dictate that she be relieved and transferred to other duties.

Therapeutic abortions are entirely legal and so are all other operations designed to save a mother's life or health. But what if an operation is not legal? Obviously if it is clearly a criminal operation, the nurse should not consent to serve. At the same time the nurse should not be too hasty at jumping to the conclusion that an operation is illegal. Custom is gradually giving more latitude to physicians so that they may use their discretion in some borderline cases, and progress certainly lies in this direction. So the nurse can very well leave such matters to the judgment of the doctor.

(4) We have already considered as an introductory example the rule of *telling the truth*. So we need add little to that here. Situations differ as to the danger of making exceptions to the rule of truthfulness. For example, accuracy in keeping hospital records is so important that it is hard to conceive of a justifiable exception. Honesty here should be so meticulous that the nurse will not even take the liberty of making an entry on a chart just a few minutes before she intends to do the thing recorded. She may be called away unexpectedly and not have an opportunity to inform the nurse who takes her place that the task has not been done. It is better to play absolutely safe in all such matters.

It would be foolish, however, to say to nurses or anybody else, "Never lie" or "Never even use deception," when we know perfectly well that there are situations which human beings will meet by some sort of deception regardless of what morality tells them. So we might as well make our ideal come within the range of human nature and admit that occasionally lying is permissible. In fact, if the harm which would come to a patient or to an institution from telling the truth is *much* greater than the harmful by-products of lying, then it is not only permissible not to tell the truth but it is one's duty not to do so.

Especially when good men or women may circumvent bad or unreasonable ones by lying there is a strong temptation to do it. Somehow in every institution there are persons of petty minds who constantly make others unhappy by too literal an interpretation of rules, or there are those who perversely or selfishly block progress. When strict truthfulness would only play into their hands, there is justification for deception, provided that it is not carried too far and that it does not become habitual and destroy the bonds of confidence upon which any institution depends.

An illustration of justifiably thwarting a fanatical and heartless person through deceit is familiar to all who have read Victor Hugo's *Les Misérables*. Jean Valjean, an escaped convict, who had originally been put in prison for stealing a loaf of bread to keep his mother from starving, has risen to a position of wealth and honor and is noted for his benefactions. Yet Javert, a detective who can think only of his duty to track down criminals, continues to hound Jean Valjean throughout his life. On one occasion, Jean Valjean is concealed by some nuns to whom he has made large gifts for charity, and when Javert appears and demands to know whether he is on the premises, one of the sisters pauses a moment, makes her decision, and lies in order to save him. Victor Hugo remarks that he is sure that that lie is recorded as a merit for her in Heaven, and most of us, we are sure, will agree with him.

One always has the feeling, however, that in admitting that deception is occasionally justifiable, we set loose in the world a dangerous principle. On the other hand, the rule of fanatically telling the truth regardless of the consequences seems even more dangerous. So we must run the risk of some evil in either choice. About the best we can do is to mitigate the possible evils connected with sanctioning white lies by concluding with this warning: You are playing with fire when you tamper with the rule of truthfulness and only a very wise person can do this without getting hurt.

(5) *Regard confidence as sacred.* Common sense tells us that that is a good rule anywhere throughout life, but in caring for the sick it is especially important because many persons when ill are not mentally normal and they frequently say things they would ordinarily suppress. One of the services due the sick and their relatives is to give them a sense of assurance that their affairs will not become public property as a result of calling in a nurse or going to a hospital. For more than two thousand years, since the formulation of the Oath of Hippocrates, physicians have adhered to the rule:

> All that may come to my knowledge in the exercise of my profession or in daily commerce with men, which ought not to be spread abroad, I will keep secret and never reveal.

And such silence is an equally sacred obligation for nurses.

And yet even here we cannot escape moral conflicts. Sometimes a patient may in confidence tell a nurse something that a physician should know—something, for example, such as the confession of an illegally induced abortion which may be of vital importance in determining prompt diagnosis and treatment. Certainly when the medical welfare of the patient thus demands it, a violation of a confidence is justifiable. Again, while nurses, like doctors, ministers, and priests, have in most cases legal immunity from divulging "privileged communications," nevertheless there may be some cases in which silence would cause so great injustice and harm to the community that the nurse would be justified in revealing even professional secrets. The public must understand that professional integrity does not mean *absolute* secrecy on the part of physicians and nurses but secrecy limited by the public welfare. It means that, "other things being equal," the patient can rely upon medical confidences being kept.

(6) One way of avoiding the strain of having one's mind loaded with too many confidences of an unnecessary sort, is to *avoid becoming intimate with patients.* "Courtesy to all but intimacy with none" might well be a slogan for nurses. In fact, in every occupation and particularly in professions it is important to keep as distinct as possible one's professional role and one's role as a private person. This does not mean that we need to

lean over backwards in maintaining a stiff formality and cold dignity and aloofness. It simply means that it is best to draw the line on intimacy somewhere this side of the place where complications of any sort may begin.

The sentiments of sick people are not very dependable and a nurse and a patient who get along famously in a hospital might not hit it off so well together in a different situation. Generally speaking, it is better for romances to develop in the area of life in which they must be lived out rather than in an abnormal, artificial situation. And yet, this rule too has exceptions, as anyone will agree who knows life and knows how few real opportunities for romance it affords, especially in occupations in which associations tend to be chiefly with those of one's own sex. So again all we can say is that the rule of professionalism usually serves the best interests of patient and nurse alike, but that in occasional instances when the rule seems to be a foolish obstacle in the way of individual happiness, only a heartless fanatic would say that the individual ought not to take a chance.

(7) *The rule against discussing religion or politics with a patient* is really a part of a broader rule which tells us that we ought not to talk about anything that upsets a patient or talk so much that he becomes fatigued. There is just the ideal amount of talk for each individual case at various stages of his recovery. Religion and politics are singled out for reference because there are still many persons who do not know how to discuss these subjects without becoming emotional and also there are some persons, who, if given half a chance, become missionaries wherever they may be. From the business standpoint alone it would be ruinous for a hospital to get the reputation of being a place where patients were annoyed by religious propaganda. And since the nurse must avoid all behavior of that sort, it is simplest just to keep shy of controversial topics altogether.

There may be instances, however, in which one can tell by the trend of the patient's conversation that a discussion of controversial subjects will have no adverse medical effects and so there is no harm in some exchange of views. Or, a little inane acquiescence does no harm now and then, provided that the nurse does not compromise her intellectual integrity too much. But, after all, it is common sense and a kind regard for the patient's welfare which must be the determining principle in each case.

(8) Both professionalism and democracy require that every patient receive the same high quality of service regardless of means. Hence it is important for the public to understand that *extra services cannot be purchased by gifts.* A patient who appreciates the dignity of the nursing profession would not insult it by the offer of a tip. There are some, however, who out of sheer gratitude would like to give some token of appreciation to a nurse. It is not easy to say what should be done in such cases. If the gift is large, obviously it should be returned with a considerate and appreciative explanation of the rule against accepting gifts. If it is small and merely symbolic, it might be the kinder thing to keep it, though with some gentle efforts to educate the patient away from such expressions of gratitude.

(9) The suggestion that *a nurse ought to be careful never to do anything for which she might be sued,* may seem more a matter of expediency than of morals. But the moral problem enters in certain emergencies in which the nurse may be impelled to do what is best for the patient even though it may involve some risk to herself. There have been cases in which patients have collected damages because some garment was torn or cut in the course of administering emergency treatment. The occasional allowance of such damages by courts probably provides a wholesome check upon the indifference of a few doctors or nurses to the property values of patients, though the motivation of such suits is frequently not honorable. In some cases, however, too great care with the patient's personal effects might involve a costly delay and the nurse may simply have to accept personal risk for the patient's sake. This is mentioned not because it is a problem that often arises but because it illustrates the sort of moral conflicts that the medical and nursing professions learn to take for granted.

(10) Nurses have not had to struggle against *commercialism* as doctors have. Nurse registries have developed in an orderly way so that there has been no problem of one nurse gaining an advantage over other nurses by being able to spend large sums in *advertising.* With physicians, however, it has been important to make advertising unethical because in the medical profession

above all others it is desirable to make success depend solely upon merit. Of course, even with advertising eliminated, there are subtle ways in which doctors with social connections or prepossessing personalities may acquire a larger practice and more wealth than equally competent colleagues. But the rule against advertising has prevented the worst abuses.

Obviously a nurse who is interested in maintaining the integrity of the medical profession and protecting the public's health will not cooperate with a physician who is engaging in unethical practices. At the same time in the present age of rapid transition from older to newer types of social institutions, nurses should learn to discriminate between truly unethical practices and progressive movements which may *seem* unethical to the conservative members of any local medical society. For example, many physicians have regarded group medicine as unfair competition. A partnership of physicians operating a clinic, with prepayment of medical fees on an annual insurance basis, has been considered a violation of the rule against contract medicine, and physicians participating in such a scheme have sometimes been expelled from medical societies and barred from hospitals. Then, in order to protect themselves and win the support of the public, some of these clinics have had to make appeals through advertising, which has further estranged them from orthodox members of the profession. Public opinion among enlightened sections of the population and the private opinion of many liberal physicians have, however, been sympathetic toward this movement in the direction of group medicine, for it has become increasingly apparent that individual medical practice has not provided adequate medical care for the middle and lower income groups.

Gradually the medical profession is changing its conception of medical ethics to make room for group practice by competent physicians with prepayment of medical fees. The rule against contract medicine was originally designed to prevent physicians from assuming contracts under which the number of patients was so large as to make proper care of them impossible. Such abuses can be prevented under group medicine if medical societies will set about the task of supervising rather than fighting this new kind of medical practice. Similarly, it is quite ethical for nurses and hospitals to cooperate with competent physicians engaging in these experiments. As long as scientific medical care is provided, with rewards to individual physicians commensurate with their abilities, that is all that ethics requires.

A word should be said about one difficult problem that nurses face because of their being on the one hand professional people who might be expected to render service whether paid for it or not and on the other hand members of a vocational group with a one-price system of charges. Not all people can pay for nursing services. Yet the nurse cannot be a self-sustained worker unless she charges for her service or unless she is a paid member of some nursing staff. The nurse cannot, if she is in private practice, charge wealthy patients more than she does others, as doctors and lawyers do. How resolve the conflict, then, between the need of the low-income classes for nursing service and the inability of the nurse to work for no salary or even for small compensation? Nurses do as a matter of fact perform a certain amount of free nursing service. For the year 1935 nurses reported an average of 11 days' service for which they were not compensated. But this is no permanent solution for the problem. One approach, which would hasten the bringing of health service to all the people, might be to arrange group nursing insurance in a manner somewhat similar to that in which group hospitalization has been provided. Surely ways must be found to bring to, the public the nursing service it needs, while at the same time assuring to nurses a secure and fair remuneration.

(11) A question that sometimes confronts the nurse, though not as frequently as it does the doctor, in her public relationships, has to do with informing the public about health matters. To what extent ought the nurse to encourage laymen to think in medical terms? On the one hand, physicians and nurses have sought to *discourage self-medication on the part of patients.* Home-doctoring usually consists in wasting money on useless and sometimes harmful patent medicines. "He who medicates himself has a fool for a patient and a fool for a physician."

On the other hand, the success of modern medicine depends upon the existence of an enlightened public. How can the nurse foster lay medical intelligence without encouraging unwise self-medication? Certain information may usually be given without question, as, for example, the stressing of essential factors related to the simple laws of personal hygiene. Interpretation to the public of such matters as adequate diet, rest, recreation, and all that makes for good health habits, is welcomed by the public and urged by most present-day physicians. Explanation regarding the meaning of immunization and the principles involved affords another example. Still another is the teaching of the public to recognize the elementary symptoms of disease and in so doing to assure care of the condition early. As important as any information the nurse may give is that stressing the need for medical examinations, particularly in the early stages of such conditions as pregnancy, tuberculosis, and venereal disease. Under our general democratic approach the tendency is growing to take the public into one's confidence as co-workers in the same cause. In fact, one of the great tasks of the good nurse is to be a reliable interpreter to the public of present-day health knowledge.

The Golden Mean

In all of the foregoing discussion we have sought to encourage a wise moderation, discrimination, and adaptability in professional conduct as opposed to a blind fanaticism in living up to rules. It is the spirit rather than the letter of the law that we have emphasized. In every case we have tried to discover the ideal point between the extremes of laxness on the one hand and rigidity on the other.

The Greek philosopher, Aristotle, over two thousand years ago worked out an entire ethics in such terms. He described most virtues as being a golden mean between two extremes. The extremes represented too much or too little of a desirable quality. In other words, there was a vice of excess and a vice of defect for each virtue. For example, courage is a virtue of which rashness or foolhardiness is the vice of excess and cowardice is the vice of defect. For the virtue of truthfulness the vice of excess is tactlessness and the vice of defect, deceitfulness. And so on. The problem is to learn how to draw the line somewhere between the two extremes in each case.

There are many personal virtues which are vital to human

happiness in all walks of life and they are perhaps even more important in the nursing profession since character and personality cannot be separated from efficiency in the service which the nurse performs. Then, too, in recent years the public has

Vice of Defect	Virtue	Vice of Excess
Cowardice	Courage	Foolhardiness
Deceitfulness	Truthfulness	Tactlessness
Dishonesty	Honesty	Over-scrupulousness
Suspiciousness	Trustfulness	Gullibility
Unfairness or Favoritism	Justice or Impartiality	Fanaticism
Stinginess	Generosity	Being "generous to a fault"
Selfishness	Unselfishness	Letting oneself be imposed upon
Cruelty or Hard-heartedness	Kindliness	Sentimentalism
Intolerance	Tolerance	Lack of discrimination
Disloyalty	Loyalty	Blind loyalty
Disobedience	Obedience	Docility
Lawlessness	Law-observance	"Leaning over back-wards"
Improvidence	Thriftiness	Miserliness
Impatience	Patience	Being too long-suffering
Irascibility	Good Nature	Lack of "spunk"
Pettiness	Magnanimity	Being too forgiving
Servility or Obsequiousness	Independence	Obstinacy or Boorishness
Weakness	Determination	Relentlessness or Importunateness
Boastfulness	Modesty	Self-depreciation
Inferiority Feeling	Self-Confidence	Conceit
Meanness or Lack of Dignity	Dignity	Haughtiness or Pomposity
Impudence, "Brass," "Crust," or "Nerve"	Reserve or Good Breeding	Shyness
Vulgarity	Refinement or Good Taste	Prudishness or Squeamishness
Aloofness	Friendliness	Promiscuousness
Self-indulgence	Temperance	Asceticism
Frigidity	Sex-normality	Voluptuousness
Laziness	Industry	Inability to relax

come to idealize nurses and expects more of them than of ordinary persons. Time, however, does not permit a discussion of the numerous virtues that make up a good character and promote a happy community. We shall have to content ourselves with simply listing a score or more of virtues in the Aristotelian manner, with their corresponding vices. Reflection upon these or discussion of them will have to be left to the student or the class.

Cooperation

Many of the moral conflicts with which we have dealt in this chapter have had to do with the relation of nurse and physician. A word in conclusion should be said about the growing cooperation between these two professions as well as other allied arts.

The Doctor. The relationship between the nurse and the medical profession has been not unlike that which has obtained in the family. The father hitherto has been the titular head of the household. But the trend in recent years has been for autocratic dictation in the family to give way to cooperative democratic endeavor. So in the medical family. The doctor and his co-workers have the common objective of the welfare of humanity. The doctor accepts chief responsibility for certain phases of this care. He it is, for example, who makes the diagnosis and prescribes the treatment. But he works cooperatively with others in the medical science field—with dietitians, technicians, pharmacists, and nurses, as they in turn work with him and with each other.

All have regard for the dignity and worth of the others. The doctor is not a lone worker, albeit the most highly trained. His service depends for its greatest effectiveness upon that of others. Does he wish to give a patient a transfusion? The nurse sets up the apparatus and assists in the administration of the treatment. Is he at a loss for knowledge concerning a patient who has suffered a stroke? The nurse's observation of the onset of the attack may be of great aid in his diagnosis and treatment. Has he need that a patient coming up for an operation be more emotionally stable? The sensitive nurse will send to the operating room a patient who is calm, trusting, and reassured. The nurse, who assists with the transfusion, who observes the onset of a stroke, who reassures the patient, is cooperating with the doctor toward the common aim of service to the patient, as she cooperates with allied workers and they with her to this same end.

The Nursing Profession. Lastly, let us touch briefly on the relationship of the nurse to her own profession. This depends largely on what she herself brings to the profession, in accordance with the truism—"Give to the world the best you have, and the best will come back to you." In relation to one's fellow workers the one thing most to be desired is a spirit of genuine interest in them, of helpfulness toward them, of appreciation for their contributions and of fine loyalty to them as co-workers in a great calling. Above all things, the perpetuation of the ideals of service for which both the nurse and her fellow workers stand is a paramount desideratum. These ideals have become crystallized in the profession of nursing itself. To a profession which has humanized its work to the point where its "native material"—"blood, vile odors, bad hours, and nervous strain"*—has become dignified and creative, to such a profession we owe much. To give our best service as individuals is admirable; to give this with a spirit of mutual understanding is commendable; but to offer the service with consciousness of cooperative contribution through an entire profession is ideal.

Study Questions

1. What three classes of persons should be served by a professional code of ethics?
2. Why is it that nurses agree, for the most part, as to borderline cases of rules in which exceptions should be made, even though each nurse has only her own vague feelings to depend upon in making up her mind?
3. What two types of consequences ought a nurse to keep in mind when deciding a difficult case of ethical conduct? Mention some of the bad consequences of lying.
4. Go through the list of eleven rules enumerated at the beginning of this chapter and think of cases in which it might be justifiable to make an exception.
5. Read through the list of virtues in the latter part of the chapter and try to think of persons or instances of conduct that illustrate the various virtues and vices. Then cover up the columns containing the two extremes and

---

* T. V. Smith: "The Democratic Way of Life," p. 162. The University of Chicago Press. 1939.

see whether you can name the vice of defect and the vice of excess for each virtue. If you think of a name that means approximately the same as the terms listed in the text, that is satisfactory.

6. What is the more modern conception of the professional relation between physician and nurse?

Questions for Thought and Discussion

1. Do you think the nursing profession ought to have a written code of ethics, as the medical profession does? Give all the arguments you can think of on both sides of this question.

2. Discuss a situation from your own experience in nursing in which these two rules conflicted with each other: (1) "Tell the truth." (2) "Don't betray confidences." In handling this situation, to which rule did you subscribe? Should the rule to tell the truth always take precedence over the rule not to betray confidences? or vice versa?

3. Discuss a situation from your own experience in nursing in which these two rules conflicted with each other: (1) "Always do what is best for the patient." (2) "Carry out the doctor's orders." Would it always be best for the patient if the nurse carried out written orders to the letter?

4. You are on duty in a hospital ward. The doctor asks you in the presence of the patient to do a treatment (for example, start an intravenous infusion) which it is contrary to hospital regulations for a nurse to carry out. How would you handle this situation? What loyalty do you owe to the doctor? to the hospital?

5. Would a code of ethics for the nursing profession help you to decide your action in the situations described in questions 2, 3, and 4? Even if you had a code of ethics, would you still have to make some choices between conflicting rules, or conflicting loyalties?

Books to Read

Cabot, Richard C.: *Adventures on the Borderlands of Ethics.* New York. Harper. 1926.

Cook, Sir Edward Tyas: *The Life of Florence Nightingale.* London. Macmillan. 1914.

Harriman, Philip Lawrence, Greenwood, Lela Lorene and Skinner, Charles Edward: *Psychology in Nursing Practice.* New York. Macmillan. 1942.

Shaffer, L. F.: *The Psychology of Adjustment.* Boston. Houghton-Mifflin. 1936.

Taeusch, C. F.: *Professional and Business Ethics.* New York. Henry Holt. 1926. Chapter VI.

XIII

Some Problems of Life and Death

The nurse, whose office it is to give comfort always regardless of whether or not she can heal, will often go with her patient down into the Valley of the Shadow. There is no substitute, as a preparation for such an experience, for personal warmth and professional idealism. This chapter will not pretend to offer one. Instead it will take up briefly and objectively a few contributions that ethics has made historically to the problems of death and some modern trends in connection with it.

The questions which are, have been, and possibly always will be asked in the presence of death are fairly constant. They may be phrased simply:

1. If this is the end for me, will all my plans and desires come to naught?

2. If this is the end for me, what will happen to those who are dependent upon me?

3. How can I adjust myself to the loss of some relative or friend?

4. Is it ever right to deprive other human beings of life?

5. Is there any limit to my duty to take risks in the service of others?

The Prospect of One's Own Death.

The question of one's own death was the subject of much speculation in the ancient Mediterranean civilizations. How should one look forward to his own demise? A great many of the ancients who were preoccupied with this question were unable to conquer their own fears. But some men did.

Pessimism. First, there were the pessimists. The pessimists concentrated their attention upon the evils of life. They kept thinking about plagues, taxes, injustice, the frailties of old age, war, and what not, until death acquired the visage of a savior. Silenus was such a pessimist, and when Midas asked him what was the best fate for man, he replied: "Pitiful race of a day, children of accidents and sorrow, why do you force me to say what were better left unheard. The best of all is unobtainable— not to be born, to be nothing. The second best is to die early." Pessimism may seem absurd to us, but there are human beings today, as there were in ancient times, to whom pessimism is entirely convincing. Having seen a great deal of trouble, they can say with the fabulous Irishman: "Sure, and it's only the hope of dying that keeps me alive."

Belief in Immortality. The second ancient position with reference to death was a strong belief in immortality. Classical civilization produced a number of new religions which were founded on faith in continued existence after natural death. The most successful of these religions was Christianity. One of the acknowledged strengths of the Christian system has always been that its teaching of immortality enables its followers to face death with assurance.

Stoicism. The third view of death was that of the Stoics. We have already considered the Stoic ideal of serene living (in Chapter X). In the presence of death, as in the presence of all other disturbances, the Stoic kept reminding himself that what he prized most was dignity, rationality, honor, and virtue. In order that he might maintain these attitudes, a Stoic like the Emperor Marcus Aurelius was ready to acquiesce in any external change. If immortality was denied to man, the Universe must have it so. "Whatever harmonizes with Thee, harmonizes with me," wrote the Stoic Emperor in his prayer to the Universe.

Epicureanism. Finally, there were Epicurus and Lucretius, who said simply, "When we are, death is not; when death is, we are not." Disbelieving in any life, good or bad, beyond the grave, they denied, with great vehemence, that our own death presents any problem at all.

Although Schopenhauer has given an eloquent exposition of the Pessimist's welcome to death, and although the other three views have received modern support, modern philosophy and theology have added little that is original to the interpretation of life's ending. The reason for this is that modern thinkers have been less occupied with the prospect of their own annihilation. They have expressed the outlook of a civilization that was interested in life. Most of the original thinking of the last three centuries has been concerned with the kind or quality of life.

Effects of Bereavement

If the best thinkers of modern times have been relatively indifferent as to what happens to the dead, we must not suppose that they have been unconcerned about mortality. They have been very much interested in what happens to the survivors. The effects of bereavement have received extensive study. Few other events have so profound an effect upon the happiness or misery of the living, and the modern, with his interest in increasing happiness and preventing misery, is anxious that the best scientific knowledge be actually used in mitigating the sorrow of bereavement.

Modern Attitude Toward Bereavement. The trend is toward those customs which help the bereaved to adjust themselves to their loss. It is violently away from those which, coming out of pre-history, tend to accentuate their grief. Gone, or on the way out, are the misery-creating usages. In many communities it is no longer required that funeral services shall be long and full of heart-rending music. The family is not expected to wear mourning clothes and isolate itself for months or years, refraining from all normal enjoyments. Widows and widowers are not severely criticized if they marry again. Irreparable as the loss may be, the losers are not held to a routine that will continually remind them of their sorrow. They are encouraged to make new associations and develop new interests.

Recognizing the increasing interdependence of mankind, people have been turning their attention to practical ways of forestalling the calamities of bereavement. To date, the most marked success along this line has had to do with provisions for economic security. Perhaps the earliest efforts to secure survivors against poverty were the unrelenting pursuit of private fortunes by breadwinners. Within the last century this has been supplemented or replaced by insurance. One no longer hears the old argument that life insurance is gambling or encroaching upon divine providence. Insurance is recognized as a sound measure for distributing the risks of life, the risks that are unpredictable for individuals but predictable for large groups. And, within the last generation, public opinion, realizing that individuals may be uninsurable or too negligent or poor to buy protection, has sanctioned a social security program, some measures of which are already attained. First came compulsory industrial accident and health insurance; later mothers' pensions and other aid to dependent children; and still later, old age pensions. Today the program, still growing and still far from completion, represents the direction of present day thought in dealing with the effects of bereavement.

The nurse who attends the hopeless case is often a great strength to the family through the control, as well as through the kindness and sympathy she shows, as she faces their trouble with them. Sometimes she can go further by asking what (constructively) can be done to relieve the hardships of the family. Does the survivor know how to notify the insurance company? What social security benefits are available? It is not the duty of the nurse to give legal or financial advice, but if she is asked, she may as a friend in need offer suggestions.

Controversial Questions

Modern society at the time of the writing of this book exhibits a number of trends which defy precedent in connection with control over life and death. In presenting these trends the authors recognize two facts about social progress. First, that progress goes by waves which advance and retreat, so that one must beware of judging by the crest of the wave how far we have actually come; and, second, that the wave bears flotsam and wreckage as well as good ships to shore. Without being sure as to the true extent or permanent beneficence of the trends, we mention the issues as questions pertinent to ethics and medicine. Six will be considered: capital punishment, warfare, martyrdom, euthanasia, contraception, and abortion.

Capital Punishment

Capital punishment has the sanction of tradition behind it as well as the weight of accepted systems of criminal justice. The questioning of it stems from humane feeling and from psychological and sociological findings about criminology. The humane person finds his feeling of the sacredness of life violated; ordinarily, however, he tells himself the violation is unavoidable if law and order are to be maintained. The case against capital punishment, however, has been put most strongly by those who question the right of the state to take life and who do not admit that the violation of the sanctity of human life is unavoidable. The writings of Emma Goldman, Proudhon, Kropotkin, and Bakunin express this point of view.

If we turn to the latest treatises on criminology we shall find many plans for preventing crime and some suggestions for substituting other measures than sheer coercion in the treatment of criminals. The problems involved reach into social conditions. Crime-breeding sections of our cities are studied; programs of housing and youth organization are advanced and carried on. It is a strong trend of our time, and its aim is to substitute prevention of the crime for punishment after it.

Warfare

Perhaps no other question than that of war can so well illustrate the fluctuation of the waves of public feeling in regard to a custom which the race is trying to outgrow. In the years between World Wars I and II pacifism made great headway. Then came the bombings of London and Pearl Harbor and pacifism receded.

Possibly a fair statement of the strong currents of mass feeling which center around this question in the western hemisphere would include the following points. First, that ethically there can be no doubt that war is bad. Second, that war is yet better than the evils of unjust aggression. And, third, in addition to the duty every right minded person has to resist aggression, there is also the duty he has to work for prevention of war.

In other words, there can be no question that in a perfect society no one should take up arms against another human being. But we do not live in a perfect society. As Grotius pointed out in his famous *De Jure Belli ac Pacis*, there continue to be disputes between nations which we are not wise enough or virtuous enough to settle peacefully, and from time to time there are inequitable encroachments. At the same time the ethical feeling of the moment seems to be a positive obligation to share in movements to preserve peace once won. This may be seen in the almost unanimous support accorded the United Nations organization in the Senate of the United States in 1945 as contrasted with the rejection of the League of Nations pact a quarter of a century earlier.

Martyrdom and Sacrificial Heroism

Martyrs are persons who voluntarily accept the risk of death rather than refrain from attempts to advance a cause in which they believe. In the history of western civilization the list of martyrs is very long indeed: Socrates, Jesus, Justin, Perpetua, Joan of Arc, Servetus, John Huss, Sir Thomas More, Elijah Lovejoy, and Edith Cavell. Tens of thousands have been martyrs for religion, for freedom of thought, for science, for the anti-slavery cause, for economic and political justice, and for country. Has this voluntary sacrifice of life been moral?

In view of the fact that human beings have martyred themselves for the sake of diametrically opposed causes, it is impossible to justify the *wisdom* of all martyrs. Nevertheless, there has never been much questioning of the martyrs' *right* to risk their lives for the sake of their causes. Common sense will concede that there may be times when other values are greater than the value of continued existence. Although we may hope for the establishment of sufficient freedom of speech so that men and women will no longer have to die in advocacy of their beliefs, we cannot deny that in the absence of that freedom the voluntary choosing of martyrdom may be justified.

Risking One's Life in Medical Research. Serious sacrifice involving risk of life is not asked of many nurses, except in time of war. Some nurses, however, face the question of hazard incident to the performance of professional duty even in peace time. The experimental stages of x-ray and radium therapy, as well as pioneer work in the control of yellow fever and other communicable diseases, called for death-dealing risks on the part of both physicians and nurses. There is no reason to believe that all dangerous experimentation is in the past. Furthermore, the acceptance of duty in certain pestilential regions or anywhere during an epidemic implies a willingness to shorten one's life. War service is certainly not the only service that is attended by unusual peril.

A rational ethics could scarcely endorse recklessness in the incurring of risks. Living dangerously just for the experience puts a greater premium on thrills than upon life, and that seems to be inverting the scale of values. Much of a nurse's education consists of lessons about precautions and the recognition of unnecessary chance-taking. A perennial item on the agenda of professional associations is the elimination of occupational hazards. Life may be sacrificed, but life should be sacrificed only for something that is worth while.

Not only nurses and physicians, but the members of many other hazardous occupations also, tacitly assume, if they do not openly declare, that the doing of their work is worth the sacrifice of some lives. If everyone sought the safest places and the least dangerous types of work, the life of our entire society would soon be in jeopardy. Beyond a certain point, the regarding of life as something to be preserved at all costs has been self-defeating.

Euthanasia

Most opposed to precedent is the question of the ethics of euthanasia. The word means literally "dying well," and is popularly known as "mercy-killing." There are two varieties of euthanasia: voluntary and involuntary. The voluntary, which is another name for suicide performed with the aid of a physician, has as its defense the aim of escaping useless suffering in the last stages of a fatal illness. It has no legal recognition, and its advocates recognize the danger of possible abuses in the practice. Involuntary euthanasia refers to the practice of destroying deformed and mentally defective children or putting to death hopelessly insane or diseased adults who are incapable of exercising judgment.

Voluntary Euthanasia. In 1939 the Gallup Poll found that 46 per cent of those interviewed were in favor of legalizing euthanasia for suffering incurables. In England, where the subject has been discussed much more than in America, the percentage in favor of voluntary euthanasia was even greater

(69 per cent). Eminent English clergymen in recent years, including Dean Inge and Dean Matthews of St. Paul's Cathedral, have signed statements approving euthanasia and affirming that it is in accord with Christian ethics.

Involuntary Euthanasia. If approximately half of the people interviewed have come to favor euthanasia for adults, we may be sure that even a larger percentage would favor putting deformed infants to death, for there is, of course, always the possibility that the diagnosis of an incurable disease in an adult may prove mistaken, while there can be no doubt in the case of a highly defective child. As an illustration of this point of view a passage may be quoted from an article by Dr. Foster Kennedy in Collier's Magazine, May 20, 1939, "To Be or Not to Be." After voicing his objections to voluntary euthanasia for adults he says:

> But the case is far different with nature's mistakes; here the brain, damaged beyond repair, perhaps in birth, life's first hazard, lacks power to grow. Here there can be, after five years of life, no error in diagnosis, nor any hope of betterment even to near normality. Nor is there mind enough to hold any instillation of a dream to live by; no hope either of normal dying. To these unfortunates we surely might be allowed legally to grant a dreamless and unending sleep.
>
> But many may say: "But these creatures have immortal souls." To them I would answer, in all respect and reverence, that to release that soul from its misshapen body which only defeats in this world the soul's powers and gifts is surely to exchange, on that soul's behalf, bondage for freedom.
>
> It would be wrong to narrate here the sad procession of these deformities—on the outskirts of every community are kind institutions where their hopeless care is wearily carried on. A week ago there came a man of forty bringing his idiot girl of four, unable to sit up or speak. She would follow a light and look toward a sound—and that was all. The heart and lungs and digestion were perfect. With such care as he gave her she might live seventy years. The mother's

absence from the clinic was explained by her having had to go back to work, for she could make more on full time for the household than could her carpenter husband who could only get work three days a week. So they'd swapped jobs and he—flabby in body and dulled in spirit—stayed home to mind what he called "the baby."

Asked if a neighbor woman couldn't help him, he said quite simply and without resentment, "No, they won't touch an idiot." He'd tried to find full-time work but in his search, he had to take the child along with him—and, "When they see the look of her, there's nothing doing."

So these fine folk are hopeless and on a cleft stick. It was possible to set them in the way of eventually having their futile burden taken care of in a charitable place, but they'll feel their contribution must always be paid, and on all their holidays and Sundays these two people will lower their value to each other by trudging wearily to see, without benefit to any, what should not be seen at all.

Opposition to Euthanasia. As we observed at the outset, public opinion is divided on the subject of euthanasia. Medical opinion is also divided. The view cited is opposed by such men as Dr. Henri Coutard of the Curie Institute and Dr. Max Cutler. The opposition comes from two sources. First, there are those who insist that mercy-killing is intrinsically a wrong act regardless of its effect on human happiness. Second, there are those who doubt whether physicians can distinguish the hopeless cases from the others, or else they are afraid that "euthanasia" will be used as a disguise for the unscrupulous taking of life. In the article quoted above Dr. Kennedy agrees with this objection to voluntary euthanasia for adults but does not believe that it is justified in regard to euthanasia for defective children. It is not clear at present just what the prevailing view of physicians will be regarding this difficult question.

Planned Parenthood

It seems certain that planned parenthood is definitely a part of the wave of the future. Two matters widely discussed in connection with it have in the last three or four decades come to be storm centers of strongly conflicting opinions in medical circles as well as with the public at large. They are contraception and abortion. It would be best to define with some care the status of each question and its relationship to planned parenthood.

As to planned parenthood (which does not imply or require contraception), practically all ethical leaders are in favorable agreement. It is accepted that it is permissible for married couples to space their children and to limit the number of their children. Polls conducted by Dr. Gallup and by the *Ladies' Home Journal* show that a large majority of the American public agree that parents should exercise intelligent control over the birth of children so that they will be born at a desirable time and so that the health of the mother as well as the economic status of the family can be protected.

Agreement on Spacing Children. It may come as a surprise to some of our readers that there is in the United States today no substantial opposition to the spacing and limiting of children. A generation ago Margaret Sanger, R.N., was not only denied the right to disseminate contraceptive information but sometimes was not allowed the privilege of holding meetings to discuss the desirability of birth control by any method.* At the present time the desirability of limiting procreation is admitted by the Catholic clergy as well as by the clergy of many other churches and the leaders of other professions.†

Since there is a popular misconception of the Catholic posi-

* See Margaret Sanger, *My Fight for Birth Control*. New York. Farrar and Rinehart. 1931.

† Moral support has been given to the birth control movement by the:
    American Unitarian Association
    Central Conference of American Rabbis
    Federal Council of Churches of Christ in America (Committee on Marriage and the Home)
    General Council of Congregational and Christian Churches
    Lambeth Conference of Anglican Bishops (London) in which the American Episcopal Church was represented
    Methodist Episcopal Church (New York Eastern Conference and Pacific Northwestern Conference)
    Presbyterian Church in the United States (Commission on Marriage, Divorce and Remarriage)
    Protestant Episcopal Church of America
    Society of Friends (Women's Problems Group)
    Universalist General Convention

tion, it may be well to quote Father Francis J. Connell. Writing in the *Atlantic Monthly*, he declared:

> The Catholic Church does not teach that married couples are obliged, or even always counseled, to have as large a progeny as is physically possible. Reasons of health or of economy not infrequently make it advisable for a couple not to have more children.*

Dom Thomas Verner Moore says that in coming to a decision on the limitation of offspring one must consider:

> The financial situation. Can the family income with such help as may be reasonably expected adequately feed, clothe, and educate another child?
>
> The character of former children. If, for example, previous children are deaf mutes and idiots, parents should refrain from having further children.
>
> The illness of the mother which might make pregnancy a serious complication.†

Koch-Preuss, an authority on Catholic ethics, states that "Broadly speaking, married couples have not the right to bring into the world children whom they are unable to support, for they would thereby inflict a grievous damage upon society."‡

Disagreement over Contraception. The status of planned parenthood, then, is secure. If for this term, however, we substitute its actual synonym, birth control, there arises acrimonious controversy. The reason is that the latter term has been connected in the popular mind with one particular method of control, the status of which is a different matter: that is, birth control is popularly identified with the use of contraceptives. In the opinion of the Catholic clergy, for instance, the proper means of limiting offspring is continence (permanent continence or periodic continence). They object to the mechanical and chemical contraceptives which have been invented to prevent conception.

* "Birth Control: The Case for the Catholic," *Atlantic Monthly*, October, 1939.

† Thomas Verner Moore, *Principles of Ethics*. Philadelphia. Lippincott. Nursing, 1937, p. 218.

‡ *A Handbook of Moral Theology*, p. 472, quoted by Leo J. Latz, *The Rhythm of Sterility and Fertility in Women*, pp. 119–120. The Latz Foundation, Chicago, 1932.

Some opposition to contraceptives has been based upon ineffectiveness or health hazards in their use. The American Medical Association would seem to have recognized such opposition and to have adopted a program for protecting the public against the harmful and unreliable. At its annual convention in June, 1937, it voted to treat birth control as a phase of preventive medicine. Specifically, the Association decided (1) to inform physicians about their medical rights in prescribing contraceptives; (2) to carry on research in materials and methods for the prevention of conception, with a view to spreading reliable information among physicians; (3) to promote thorough instruction in medical schools in the positive and negative aspects of human fertility; and (4) to bring all dispensaries and clinics under legal licensure and medical control.

The opposition to contraception is not, however, founded upon utilitarian considerations. While admitting the desirability of limiting offspring, the opponents declare that revelation and reason specifically brand the use of contraceptives as sinful. Once more, this time in deciding the morality of contraception, we must make up our minds whether there are any actions which are absolutely and eternally right or wrong, or whether the rightness of an act depends upon the contribution which it makes to human welfare.

Abortion

Of still another status, legally, as well as in medical, ecclesiastical, and the public regard, is the practice of abortion. The same conflict between utilitarian and absolute ethics, however, appears in connection with this problem. Catholic doctrine will again be considered as representing the approach of absolute ethics to the problem. According to Catholic tradition, a direct attack upon an innocent life is held to be wrong. The only grounds upon which a human life may be taken are: (1) the protection of society against criminals; (2) self-defense against an unjust aggressor; and (3) extreme necessity (presumably covering cases of an innocent but insane person running amuck, unless such cases might be classified as unjust, though innocent, aggression). Because the unborn fetus is not guilty of the enumerated offenses, anyone who causes the fetus to be destroyed and expelled from the womb is adjudged guilty of murder. Circumstances and consequences are not considered. The sole question is whether the abortionist intends to destroy the fetus.

This method of moral reasoning can be brought into clearer light by considering a border-line case: the ectopic pregnancy. In such a case the fertilized egg cell develops in one of the fallopian tubes instead of descending into the uterus and imbedding itself there in the normal way. When the embryo reaches a certain size the tube will be ruptured and the resulting hemorrhage is likely to cost the mother's life. Hence, the usual procedure is to operate as soon as the ectopic pregnancy is discovered. A direct assault upon the life of the embryo, however, would be contrary to Catholic ethics and most Catholic moralists have hitherto held that all that could be done was to wait until the hemorrhage began and then operate—after the embryo was presumably dead—which would, in most cases, be too late to save the life of the mother. Dom Thomas V. Moore, however, in his *Principles of Ethics* (p. 169) advocates immediate operation when the ectopic pregnancy is discovered. He says that Catholic morality justifies attacking the threat of hemorrhage in the tube by clamping the arteries. Shutting off the blood supply will, of course, cause the death of the embryo, but since this is *incidental* to the attack upon the abnormal condition of the tube, it is not considered wrong.

In Catholic textbooks we find that moral conclusions depend upon (a) whether an act is considered intrinsically evil and (b) whether an evil consequence is a product of the immediate primary intention or not. Thus, there are a few cases where the destruction of the fetus is allowed incidentally to the saving of the mother's life. If, for example, a cancer of the uterus is discovered in the course of a pregnancy, the entire uterus may be removed, resulting of course in the death of the fetus. In that case, the physician's immediate primary intention is presumed to be the removal of the cancerous tissue and not the destruction of the fetus. On the other hand, abortion induced because of heart disease, tuberculosis or nephritis (a kidney disease) is immoral according to Catholic doctrine because the taking of the life of the fetus is direct rather than incidental.

Medical Attitude toward Abortion. According to Norman E. Himes, most medical textbooks approve of abortion in the case of heart disease, tuberculosis, and nephritis. Furthermore, he says:

> Leading authorities on abortion are ready to grant that in addition to the above conditions, women who are mentally defective or psychologically irresponsible (as in the case of a woman who becomes pregnant during the manic stage of a manic-depressive psychosis), or girls on whom incest or rape has been performed, are entitled to an abortion. Likewise a woman who seriously threatens suicide in the event that her pregnancy is not terminated should be aborted. This is the view of many experts on the matter, though it might not be supported as yet by the majority of physicians. Liberal doctors, furthermore, would include not only all of the above cases but add those of extreme poverty accompanied by physical depletion, while a few would go even further and include instances involving illegitimacy, desertion and widowhood.*

The physician and those most vitally concerned would be allowed to decide upon an abortion if circumstances clearly indicated anguish or want would result from the birth of a child. A recent amendment of the abortion law in Sweden allows physicians just such discretion. They are allowed to perform abortions for "humanitarian" reasons, e.g., in instances of rape or for eugenic reasons or for "mixed medical-social" reasons. As yet in the United States and most other countries abortions are legal only when performed to protect the life or health of a pregnant woman.

Study Questions

1. What were the four ancient philosophies regarding death?
2. What changes have occurred in customs regarding bereavement?
3. What are the practical problems which are created by bereavement?

* Norman E. Himes, and Abraham Stone, *Practical Birth Control Methods*, pp. 160–161. New York. Viking Press. 1942.

4. What are the arguments pro and con in regard to the use of force against criminals? In war?
5. How far should one go in risking death for the sake of some cause?
6. What percentage of the public in England and America favor laws legalizing voluntary euthanasia? Have any Christian ministers expressed approval?
7. On what grounds is euthanasia opposed?
8. What does the Gallup Poll reveal concerning the attitude of the American public toward the morality of birth control, or planned parenthood?
9. State the recent attitude of Catholic moralists toward the intelligent control of the birth of children.
10. What decisions did the American Medical Association reach regarding contraception in 1937?
11. On what grounds is contraception advocated and opposed?
12. When is it permissible to take a human life, according to Catholic morality?
13. What is the Catholic attitude toward causing death of an embryo incidentally in the case of disease? Show how Dom Thomas V. Moore applies Catholic principles in such a way as to save the lives of mothers where possible within the framework of Catholic ethics.
14. When is abortion legal in the United States? What suggestions does Dr. Himes make for liberalizing abortion laws?
15. What approach would utilitarian morality make toward the problems of euthanasia, contraception, and abortion?

Questions for Thought and Discussion

1. Do you believe that departments of public health should concern themselves about providing contraceptive advice for poor parents, as has been done in North Carolina, South Carolina, and Alabama? Give reasons for your view.
2. Do you believe that there should be social reforms that would make it possible for poor people, who are phys-

ically fit and want to have children, to rear and educate a family properly?

3. Ought public health nurses teach poor mothers how to prevent conception or should they confine themselves to referring cases to private physicians or clinics?

4. Should nurses advise parents concerning problems of numbers and spacing of children, even though the parents have not had medical advice regarding chemical or mechanical contraceptive devices?

5. A birth rate such as existed in the United States in the thirties will not be sufficient to maintain a stable population, once the increments in population due to increased average length of life ceases. If our population should begin to decline, what do you suggest doing about it?

6. During the nineteenth century Europe served as a city for rural America, doing most of our manufacturing for us, and therefore she was able to build up a population larger than her resources could support. Now, however, we do most of our own manufacturing. Does this indicate the need of a new population policy for Europe? Is the failure of Europe to reduce her population a cause of war?

7. Do you think that abortion laws ought to be liberalized? Do you think that liberalized abortion laws would tend to reduce invalidism following abortion? How far do you think a state should go in legalizing abortion?

8. What would you say to the proposition that all persons, whether in institutions or not, should be sterilized as soon as school tests and records indicate subnormal mental ability? At what level of ability should a person be considered sufficiently subnormal to require sterilization?

9. Do you think that it should be legal for a physician to put deformed infants to death? When should a child be considered sufficiently defective for this? Should there be an age limit below which a child would not be put to death? Should there be an upper age limit, requiring that defective children be put to death *before*

reaching a specified chronological age? Should parental consent to euthanasia be required in all cases? Should the approval of more than one physician be required in each case of euthanasia? Should approval of a legally constituted medical board be required in each case of euthanasia?

10. If you were the nurse taking care of an infant and it was discovered that the child was a blind deaf-mute, would you consider that this child would be better off dead? Would you think that parents would be better off without this child? Helen Keller was a blind deaf-mute, yet she lived to become an inspiration to many persons handicapped by some physical disadvantage. Do you think that the enormous cost of educating a deaf-mute, and the devotion of the entire time of one or more persons to the care and rearing of such a child is justifiable? Give reasons for your opinion.

11. If you believe that, in general, badly deformed infants should be put to death, would you feel that exceptions should sometimes be made? If so, on what basis do you think exceptions should be made? If the practice of putting badly deformed infants to death were to be universally accepted, would there be any benefit to humanity in preserving the lives of a few such infants in order to conduct medical or other research?

12. Ought a physician to take the law into his own hands at present and see to it that a defective infant does not survive? Ought a physician to hasten the death of a person who is suffering intensely from an incurable disease? If so, which means of hastening death would you consider justifiable and which not?

13. You are a nurse taking care of a defective infant. The doctor has ordered that the infant be bottle fed using a rubber nipple. You find that the child is unable to take the formula through a nipple and the doctor does not order any other method of feeding. Would you feel that it was right to let this infant die of inanition, or would you feel that you had done wrong to remain silent? Would your attitude be the same or different

if this feeding problem involved a premature rather than a defective infant?

14. The nurse many times is in a position to make it possible for a patient to carry out the implications of his own moral code; sometimes the nurse is in a position to prevent a patient from carrying out these implications. Does the nurse who differs from a patient in her personal convictions have a responsibility to do the most in her power to help thè patient to carry out his own code?

Books to Read

Everett, Millard S.: *The Hygiene of Marriage*, rev. ed. New York. The Vanguard Press. 1942. (Also in Tower Books series.)

Himes, Norman Edwin, and Stone, Abraham: *Practical Birth-Control Methods*. New York. Viking Press. 1942.

Latz, Leo J.: *The Rhythm of Sterility and Fertility in Women*, rev. ed. Chicago. Latz Foundation. 1934.

Sutherland, Edwin H.: *Principles of Criminology*, 3rd ed. rev. Philadelphia. J. B. Lippincott Co. 1939.

XIV

Marriage and a Career

Should a nurse marry? Should she continue nursing after marriage? These are not academic questions. To many a woman they represent very real choices. Our grandmothers and most of our mothers faced no such options. The problem has arisen within the last two generations, being an outcome of the peaceful but all-encompassing revolution through which our society has been passing.

If there had been no titanic migrations or epochal inventions, if society had stood still, the old guide posts might still have been reliable. "Woman's place is in the home" might still have stood unchallenged, an unwritten but none the less strong social rule. It would have meant from one point of view shelter and, from another, limitation for the individual woman. And it would have meant the preservation of a much treasured source of idealism for society—the old-fashioned home.

Whether we like it or not, our society is in such a state of flux that tradition, appearing in the guise of an absolute morality, cannot dictate all of our choices. The lot of women is so variable that, while some succeed in living a very traditional existence, others cannot do so if they wish to. And not all of them wish to.

How often does one hear the expression: "Well, it depends upon the individual"? That expression signalizes situations in which antique customs have broken down. If there is to be any rationality in conduct in such situations, someone will have to do some thinking. Someone will have to ask how women can conduct themselves so that sanity, a reasonable amount of life's pleasures, and wholesome social relations will be secured.

Changes in Woman's Status and Work

Let us do a bit of thinking about the nurse's prospects. But before settling down to specific questions, suppose that we take a look at the larger picture, the effect of the industrial revolution and the last century's migrations on women generally.

Effect of Industrial Revolution on Women's Lives. Everyone knows about the industrial revolution. The steam engine was invented in 1764 and then came factories and cities and all of that. But does everyone *understand* the story? Understand, that is, the full effects of industry upon our own lives? Everyone knows about migrations, too. America was the refuge for the downtrodden and the haven for the oppressed. Pioneers, the melting pot: we know about that. But do we understand it?

The decisive change which has come about in the lives of women is the change in work. Women worked in the pre-industrial society of a century and a half ago, but most of them did their work at home, as members of the family group. They helped raise the food which they cooked, made clothing, gave the children what education there was, spun, wove, nursed, entertained, laundered, did everything for their homes. At that time restaurants, laundries, schools, textile mills, and clothing factories were unimportant in the lives of most people. So were canneries and packing houses, hospitals, furniture factories, hotels, theaters, and soap factories. The growth of these establishments has been simply the reverse side of the decline of household production.

By the year 1930 more than 25 per cent of the adult female population of the United States was gainfully employed away from home. More than 10 per cent of the married women were so engaged. In the professions women practically equaled men in numbers: there were 1,400,000 women in the professions, three-fifths of them teachers and one-fifth of them nurses. The depression of the thirties checked the increase in female employment, but the war boom of 1940 gave a tremendous impetus to the long-time trend. Female employment (outside of agriculture) stood at 10 million in December, 1940. One year later the figure was 12 million. Two years later it was 14 million.

The industrialization of America affected all women, not merely the 25 per cent who were in 1930 working for wages and salaries. The women who stayed at home were performing only a few of the functions which their great-grandmothers had performed. As a consequence of this leisure another problem arose, that of the capable woman who felt left out of the current of life. Many suffered the drag of too much time on their hands, and the dispiriting feeling of not being needed. Amusements, club work, and social life were only partially successful in dispelling it.

The Growth of Equality. The nineteenth century witnessed the destruction of many inequalities between the sexes, particularly in the United States. When women began to do more and more of their work away from home, they acquired many legal rights, such as the right to make wills. Some of the old inequalities in the law of divorce and the law of inheritance were removed. They were grudgingly permitted, and then encouraged, to attend school. Gradually, the disgrace of working for pay was transformed into respectability. Elizabeth Blackwell, the first female medical graduate, endured the most cruel ostracism. For three years while she was studying at Geneva, N. Y., the women at her boarding house refused to speak to her, and drew aside their skirts in contempt when they met her on the street. At the end of the century Dr. Blackwell was the subject of praise and tribute, although considerable prejudice against women physicians lingered on.

The right to vote was won, first in school elections, later in general elections. The suffragettes were met by withering ridicule, but the nineteenth amendment closed the argument at the end of the first world war. Susan B. Anthony, "the unsexed woman" who dared to speak in public, was honored on her centenary by having her picture on a postage stamp.

As a result, then, of the industrial revolution, we find the whole life picture drastically changed for women. Not only in occupation, but in legal and economic status, they faced different conditions from their mothers. An industrial and commercial technology needed women workers and needed them educated and freed from any ancient taboos. A difficulty arose from all this. There is always a cultural lag with sweeping industrial changes. In other words, people in homes throughout the country are confused in their thinking by the swift changes from old to new ideals. Added to this is the fact that a few women, sensing the possibilities and enjoying the new freedom, championed the revolution and tried to speed it up: they demanded equal rights. But millions were not so sure about "emancipation." Either they wanted to return to the good old days or they were worried about what would happen to them under the new conditions. Since the traditions of an agricultural society and even some of the traditions of a nomadic culture survived in literature, religion, law, and moral instruction, the training of girls was a mixture of incompatible ingredients.

Today many a woman finds in herself two contrary ambitions. One looks toward a career. The other looks toward a more sheltered life which is tied to the career of her husband. Thus it is that the remaining inequalities of the sexes are subjects of sharp dispute. Should women be admitted to the higher executive positions and to all of the trades and professions? Should they be admitted to any college or university? Should they receive equal pay for equal work? Should married women be given employment, particularly public employment?* Should the remaining legal inequalities be removed as in the case of guardianship rights, contractual rights, responsibility for illegitimate children, and the establishment of legal residence?

Our immediate interest is of course not the determination of public policy on these matters, but the presentation of the entire social picture, with its confused currents moving in contrary directions, as the background against which women in general and nurses in particular have to make their personal choices. The personal choices must be made. It would have been easier some generations ago. The historical trend and the public controversies, however, should be borne in mind when one is making personal decisions about one's career. It very often happens that a difference of opinion in the home or misunderstandings between parents and children or between sweethearts take on a very different appearance when viewed in the larger perspective. A difficulty that seems to grow out of some individual's mean disposition will be seen as the operation of titanic economic and cultural forces. That does not relieve the individuals

---

* During the 1930's bills were introduced into a number of state legislatures to prohibit the hiring of married women.

concerned of the necessity for making some choices, but it may help them to choose intelligently.

Must Nurses Lose Their Femininity?

Obviously, in the long periods when women occupied an economically and legally distinct position, they acquired a great many customs and manners which were quite different from the manners and characteristics of men. In the course of time these traits became almost indistinguishable from biological traits. Indeed, scientists have considerable difficulty now determining which of the sex differences are biological and which are cultural in their origin.

Not a few of the traits which helped a woman adjust to her situation in a household economy do just the reverse in an industrial economy. Consider, for example, such a patently cultural characteristic as the manner of dress. Seventy years ago Miss Anna Brackett wrote this now amusing paragraph:

> The question of woman's dress, for instance, is never to be solved by approaching it from the outside. Earnest and vigorous writers may tell women what they ought to do, and we all know perfectly well that if the skirts of our dresses ended at the tops of our boots, and we were warmly clad beneath in the full trousers proposed years ago by Mrs. Bloomer, we could take much more exercise without fatigue, and should be saved much time and much annoyance. Who but a woman can appreciate the trouble of always being obliged to use one hand in carrying her skirts up long flights of stairs? Who but a woman knows the inconvenience of her long skirts in entering or leaving a carriage, or in a strong wind? Who but a woman knows that it is utterly impossible to take even a short walk on a rainy day, however well protected, without bringing into the house an amount of wet clothing which necessitates almost an entire change? . . . For whose admiration and attraction do our young women array themselves? To please whom do they leave off their flannels and attend evening entertainments in low-necked dresses, sweep the pavements with their ornately trimmed skirts, and wear thin

boots which shall display to better advantage the well-turned foot?*

This is a revealing passage because it shows the conflict between the customs of an industrial society and those of the half-changed Mid-Victorian city. Upper class women had been relieved of their household work, but had not yet been enlisted for new duties; and so the controlling objective in clothing themselves was to secure admiration. But the practical demands of an industrial society finally changed this. Women now wear a garb more suited to their work in hospitals, offices, factories, and the centers of community activity. The kinds of clothing which, in the 1870's, seemed necessary to femininity, are now discarded. Many of the women who have made the change still seem feminine, but not in such a way as to make a career and efficient work impossible.

More subtle are the questions raised about certain feminine attitudes. A girl who, in the tradition of the Gay Nineties, faints at the sight of blood has no place in the nursing profession. Many attitudes formerly associated with women are definite liabilities. Among these are false modesty, helplessness when it comes to fixing things, excessive talking, and the tendency to take things personally.

The idea of the Golden Mean may be appropriate in taking leave of the traits with which a pre-industrial age endowed women. Certainly no patient and no colleague will welcome the nurse who on the slightest provocation bursts into tears. But that does not mean that callousness is welcomed either. As we create a culture appropriate to our age, women will develop more independent and matter-of-fact attitudes, though perhaps in the process some of them may overdo it a little.

Sex differences are changing and diminishing. By a little thought now and then we can help guide this fundamental transformation. When we think about the problem, we can recognize not one but several consequences which are to be hoped for. We want to be (1) efficient in our work, (2) natural (in the sense of not being strained or affected), (3) pleasing in

* Anna C. Brackett: *The Education of American Girls*, pp. 380–381. G. P. Putnam's Sons. 1874.

appearance and manner, and (4) sufficiently feminine to inspire true love in a worthy man. Just how these consequences can be achieved will vary with our individual inheritances, our communities and associates, and our working environments.

Should Nurses Marry?

At one time a large proportion of the nursing profession consisted of nuns who had taken the vow of celibacy. Nunneries continue to find recruits, but not in large enough numbers to maintain the nursing staffs even of Catholic hospitals. Although humanity owes a great debt to nuns, and although the system of holy orders has its advantages, the fact is that society cannot now depend upon this personnel policy in the nursing profession. The question of the marriage of nurses is, therefore, a vital one.

When to Marry? Nurses have as much right to expect matrimony as any other class of women. The steam age and the electrical age, much as they disturbed the traditional family relationships, did not destroy the family. Although divorce rates are three times as high as they were in 1880, the percentage of adults who are married is also higher than it was in 1880. Furthermore, the age at which marriage occurs has been declining during the past fifty years, particularly for men. In 1930 more than 10 per cent of the women in the fifteen to nineteen year age group were married; more than 50 per cent of the women between the ages of twenty and twenty-four were married. Nearly 75 per cent in the twenty-five to twenty-nine group and more than 80 per cent of the thirty-five to forty-four group were no longer single.* The marriage rate for all nurses less than forty years of age (48.4) is somewhat higher than for other groups of professional women.†

Since marriage has not been abolished by the gainful employment of women, two practical questions present themselves to the young nurse: When? and Who? The question about the time of marriage is partially answered by Mother Nature. If a woman wishes to bear children, she must do so before she

* Thompson and Whelpton: *Population Trends in the United States*, p. 205. McGraw Hill Book Co. 1933.
† American Journal of Nursing, vol. 42: 773.

reaches the latter forties (in some cases earlier than that). Because childbearing is much easier when the mother is young, late marriage has decided disadvantages. It is also true that the establishment of congenial parent-child relationships as well as of parent-parent relationships is easier in the twenties than in the thirties and forties. But these are not the only considerations. Economic, educational, and other factors may outweigh the child-bearing factor. Hence, there is only a presumption in favor of marriage prior to the age of thirty. In some cases, later marriage is quite sensible.

Choice of Mate. The question about the person to marry is also complex. We have already frowned upon the courtship that is allowed to develop in the line of professional duty (though there are exceptions, as we admitted in Chapter XII). The nurse's problem in finding a compatible mate is somewhat more hazardous than the average. In the first place, she gets her training and does most of her work in the city. The ratio of eligible men to eligible women is lower in nearly every city than it is in the rural regions.*

In the second place, having almost exclusively female colleagues at work and often having few out-of-work associations, nurses suffer more than some occupational groups from the segregation of the sexes. By the segregation of the sexes we mean the separation of boys and girls and later of men and women not only through the maintenance of separate schools but also by the development of different recreational and social interests. We also refer to the poverty of many communities in institutions and organizations which will give the young people a chance to get well acquainted. The traditional segregation did no harm in the days when most marriages were arranged by the parents; but now that nearly every match is made by the prospective bride and groom themselves, segregation cuts down the chances of congenial persons finding each other.

* "In the city of over a million . . . there are 133 single men to 100 single women, while in cities of 50,000 the ratio is 112." "At the ages of 20 to 30 years there are 210 single men for 100 single women on the farms." Ogburn and Nimkoff: *Sociology*, pp. 544, 525. Houghton Mifflin Co. 1940. The reason why the ratio of single men to single women is higher than 100 in every case results from the fact that women marry younger than men.

The long-run moral is to encourage customs and build up organizations that provide opportunities for young men and young women to come together for education, recreation, work, and civic activity. The short-run moral is for the nurse to avoid a shut-in life or an exclusively female companionship. Another short-run moral is to beware of the short courtship and marriage to a man who is known only as a good dancer or an obliging theater escort. There are statistics to substantiate this warning and also to indicate what factors are conducive to success in marriage. Space is lacking for a complete analysis of the statistics, and anyway the factors that would be of interest would vary with each individual. We shall merely refer the interested reader to Burgess and Cottrell, *Predicting Success or Failure in Marriage* (Prentice-Hall, Inc., 1939) and Lewis Terman, *Psychological Factors in Marital Happiness* (McGraw Hill Book Co., 1938).

When she enters the profession, a nurse obligates herself to render nursing service. Society can ill afford to waste its all too inadequate training facilities on women who have no serious intentions with respect to practicing their profession. On the other hand, the nurse does not obligate herself to forego the privileges of married life. The result is a problem: how to reconcile marriage and a career? In saying that it is a problem we do not mean that it is a subject for brooding or worrying. Brooding and worrying are not problem-solving thought. Usually they only make the problem harder. The problem calls for intelligent alertness to seize opportunities that may lead to marital happiness and for intelligent caution to recognize bad risks when opportunity presents itself.

Should Married Women Continue Nursing?

Our last question is already answered by implication in the preceding paragraphs. If a trained nurse is duty-bound to give society the benefit of her training, and if most nurses may reasonably expect marriage, the logical conclusion is that a good many married women should continue nursing. In the national survey of registered nurses made in 1943, it was found that 55.7 per cent of all nurses who responded to the survey's

questionnaire were married.* Of the active nurses answering
the questionnaire 39.6 per cent were married.†

Dilemmas. Two typical dilemmas merit discussion. First, how
can a mother follow her career and not neglect her husband and
children? Second, what should be done when the career of the
wife and the career of the husband call for residence in different
localities? It would be the height of folly to attempt to lay down
absolute rules in answer to these questions. Reasons of health,
personal idiosyncrasies, and what not, often dictate opposite
courses of action. We can only hope to dispel some proverbial
notions that seem thoughtful but often merely echo tradition
unthinkingly.

Taking the second question first, What should be done when
the career of the wife and the career of the husband call for
residence in different localities? Traditional people who like to
appear profound are apt to quote the old saw about "Out-of-
sight, out of mind." To that the sufficient reply is the equally
old saw, "Absence makes the heart grow fonder." Inanities out
of the way, it is true that physical separation is hazardous to
marriage, that is, to some marriages. We have a considerable
amount of experience to go on in the separations due to war
service and the family life of traveling men. The danger of
developing divergent interests and the danger of a triangle are
increased. But there are thousands of marriages that have with-
stood these dangers. Speaking in generalities, we can only
conclude that physical separation is to be avoided where possible, but there are many couples who have good reason to expect
such an arrangement to be successful over limited periods of
time.

When we come to the care of children, generalizations must
also be guarded and qualified. Early training and communities
being what they are, some women are probably foolish to
attempt both motherhood and a career. Of course, during an
emergency, very few nurses have an excuse for not making
temporary arrangements for the care of even small children so
that they can devote themselves to the need of the hour. Similarly, there is no particular obstacle confronting the "post-

* United States Public Health Service, 1943.
† Facts About Nursing, 1943, p. 15.

graduate mother," except perhaps a refresher course if she has been out of practice for a number of years. Another fairly easy question is part-time service which will require no more absence from home than is occasioned by the average woman's club and church work. The puzzler is full-time nursing for the mother of pre-school children.

The puzzle is not satisfactorily solved by leaving the children in charge of an ignorant maid or cleaning woman. That is unfair to the child. It may, at least temporarily, be solved by leaving the children in charge of an unemployed husband or a relative qualified to look after children. Other ways have also been found.

Nursery Schools. One way that carries much promise is the nursery school and the day nursery. Nursery schools were the fastest growing part of our educational system during the thirties. They have been much criticized. Some nurseries were and are unfit for their work. They are, however, becoming better as a class. Much of the criticism leveled at them represents a cultural lag on the part of the critics. The supply of excellently trained nursery school teachers has been increasing, and some states have a licensing system to eliminate institutions that are started by unscrupulous or ignorant persons.

The upbringing of the nursery school child compares favorably with the upbringing of the child who spends all his time at home. Performance on intelligence tests is superior.* And the development of such characteristics as curiosity, orderliness. sympathy, sociability, etc., proceeds more rapidly in the nursery school than in the home, *on the average.*† "On the average" is italicized, because the career woman's maternal responsibility does not end with the selection of a good nursery school. The progress of the child must be watched, for there are a few children who do not respond to group methods and occasionally one will encounter a child who cannot get along with a particular teacher. This admission does not invalidate the nursery school idea any more than the many failures of parents to get along with their own children invalidates the idea of home training.

* B. L. Wellman: "Effect of pre-school attendance upon the I.Q." *Journal of Experimental Education.* 1:48–69, 1932.

† Murphy and Murphy: *Experimental Social Psychology.* New York. Harper 1931, p. 316.

In good nurseries the teachers will notify the parent promptly of any maladjustment, but all too often busy parents do not pay much attention to such reports.

In this chapter we have not told you what to do. What we have tried to do is to present several problems of choice in such a way that you will plan instead of blunder, weigh consequences instead of worry, proceed thoughtfully instead of following either the line of least resistance or the line of outworn traditions. We do not believe that it is necessary for nurses to lose their femininity. We believe that most nurses should contemplate marriage. We believe that most married nurses should not call a complete and permanent halt to their professional career when they put on wedding rings. But sometimes it is easier said than done, and there are a good many practical pointers that any intelligent nurse can lose sight of in an impulsive moment.

Study Questions

1. Mention some sex inequalities in previous centuries.
2. Did women enter economic pursuits for the first time during and after the industrial revolution?
3. What sexual inequalities continue to exist? What inequalities are disappearing?
4. Why did some women fail to welcome the women's rights movement?
5. What traditionally feminine characteristics are a liability to a nurse?
6. What feminine characteristics are an asset?
7. In what age-period approximately do most women get married? Is there a best time for marrying and bearing children?
8. What difficulties may arise as a result of combining a career and marriage? How may these difficulties be overcome?
9. What can be said in favor of nursery schools?

Questions for Thought and Discussion

1. Mention some problems which might arise if a man and wife were both employed.

2. What are the advantages and disadvantages of a nurse's continuing to pursue her career after marriage?
3. Men nurses have complained that they are not given equal opportunity with women in the nursing profession. In what respects are men nurses discriminated against? Is this discrimination any more to be condoned than discrimination against women physicians and lawyers?
4. What type of nursing do you think will fit best into your own matrimonial plans?
5. How would you find out whether a prospective husband would tolerate a career on your part?
6. Think of a married woman who is following her career without domestic friction and one who has had family trouble as a result of her career. Can you analyze the two cases and spot the essential difference?

Books to Read

Burgess, Ernest W., and Cottrell, Leonard S., Jr.: *Predicting Success or Failure in Marriage*. New York. Prentice-Hall, Inc. 1939.

Ogburn, William F., and Nimkoff, Meyer F.: *Sociology*. Boston. Houghton Mifflin. 1940. Chapter XXII.

Reuter, Edward Byron, and Runner, Jessie Ridgway: *The Family*. New York. McGraw-Hill. 1938.

Terman, L. M.: *Psychological Factors in Marital Happiness*. New York. McGraw-Hill. 1938.

Tufts, J. H.: *America's Social Morality*. New York. Henry Holt. 1933. Chapters VI and XVIII.

XV

Living Democratically

W<small>HAT SHALL</small> the modern nurse think as she looks from her professional viewpoint at the social and political problems of the day?

In this and the following chapter the aim will be to present some applications of ethics to democratic living and ideals. In the last chapter we shall ask what can be done in an organized way to promote greater democracy. In this chapter the question is: "What can I do in my individual conduct to promote democracy?"

Just what is the democracy of our time? Does it differ from that of the last generation? Our answer will be taken from a declaration by the National Resources Planning Board in September of 1942:

> "We look forward to securing, through planning and cooperative action, a greater freedom for the American people. Great changes have come in our century with the industrial revolution, the acceleration of transportation and communication, the growth of modern capitalism, and rise of the national state with its economic programs. Too few corresponding adjustments have been made in our provisions for human freedom. In spite of all these changes, that great manifesto, the Bill of Rights, has stood unshaken 150 years. And now to the old freedoms we must add new freedoms and restate our objectives in modern terms:

> "F<small>REEDOM OF SPEECH AND EXPRESSION, FREEDOM TO WORSHIP, FREEDOM FROM WANT,</small> and F<small>REEDOM FROM FEAR,</small> these are the universals of human life.

> "The translation of freedom into modern terms appli-

able to the people of the United States includes, as the National Resources Planning Board sees it, the following declaration of rights:

"1. THE RIGHT TO WORK, usefully and creatively through the productive years;

"2. THE RIGHT TO FAIR PAY, adequate to command the necessities and amenities of life in exchange for work, ideas, thrift, and other socially valuable service;

"3. THE RIGHT TO ADEQUATE FOOD, CLOTHING, SHELTER, and MEDICAL CARE;

"4. THE RIGHT TO SECURITY, with freedom from fear of old age, want, dependency, sickness, unemployment, and accident;

"5. THE RIGHT TO LIVE IN A SYSTEM OF FREE ENTERPRISE, free from compulsory labor, irresponsible private power, arbitrary public authority, and unregulated monopolies;

"6. THE RIGHT TO COME AND GO, TO SPEAK OR TO BE SILENT, free from the spyings of secret political police;

"7. THE RIGHT TO EQUALITY BEFORE THE LAW, with equal access to justice in fact;

"8. THE RIGHT TO EDUCATION, for work, for citizenship, and for personal growth and happiness; and

"9. THE RIGHT TO REST, recreation, and adventure; the the opportunity to enjoy life and take part in an advancing civilization."*

The statement just quoted is worth re-reading. Crystallizing as it does recent thought about democratic aims, it is a careful summation by a responsible government agency.

The American people have a long way to go in the realization of these ideals. Indeed, some one is almost sure to say that ideals are ideals and we can never attain them. But such pessimism springs from a misunderstanding of the relation of individual citizens to their government. We can all see how in our personal dealings with people we can respect the rights of others and occasionally do a great deal to make sure that someone else gets a square deal. But as individual citizens we are inclined to feel helpless when confronted with certain gross inequalities, such

* *Post-War Planning*, p. 32. National Resources Planning Board, 1942.

as the lack of opportunities for the children of the poor or of racial minorities. Or, as individuals, we seem able to do little for the millions who do not enjoy the right to work or the right to fair pay. As the source of governmental authority and power, however, we can do much to rectify these large-scale inequalities. A hundred years ago, men like Horace Mann must have felt pretty pessimistic at times about the elimination of illiteracy. Women like Dorothea Dix must have been discouraged about the possibility of providing decent hospitals for the mentally ill. But Horace Mann and Dorothea Dix saw to it that society made an organized attack upon the evils of illiteracy and insanity. They convinced their contemporaries that the taxing power of the government should be used to finance schools and asylums, the like of which no individuals—however wealthy—could have established.

So it is in our day. To reach the objectives of democracy we must act individually and collectively. The securing of democratic rights depends in part upon our personal conduct, in part upon the activity of government and other institutions which pool our resources and good will.

How Nurses Can Promote Democracy. A nurse is frequently in a position where she can promote democracy or retard its progress. In her personal career, she meets all kinds and conditions of people, including the underprivileged. She may accept all of the existing discriminations and help to perpetuate inequalities by her unequal treatment of those with whom she comes in contact. Or, she may, as far as possible, minister to human needs regardless of ancient prejudices.

The nurse's personal attitude, however, toward patients, tradesmen, etc., is not the full extent of her contribution to democracy. Since nursing has become a full-fledged profession, its members have not only a superior technical knowledge of certain public problems but also a better general education than the average citizen. Nurses are, therefore, in a position to furnish their share of leadership in solving the many political, economic and social problems which confront us today. By voting intelligently, by expressing intelligent opinions in her conversation, and by participating in good movements, the modern nurse can frequently do her bit in speeding up the community's conquest of evils that are too much for one person to handle alone.

In this chapter we intend to discuss the more personal aspects of democracy. What is the difference between a person who lives democratically and the undemocratic person? More specifically, how can a nurse show that she is sincerely democratic?

It is fair to say that some people are undemocratic without intending to be undemocratic or even without being aware of it. Class distinctions and intolerance existed in their childhood environment and so are simply taken for granted. If you ask these people about the inequality of human rights, they will probably tell you that everyone has an opportunity in the United States. America, you will be told, is unlike the Old World: in America there are no classes; any child has a chance to be President, or if not President, a chance to make a good living and be somebody.

Inequality of Opportunity

The United States is certainly much more democratic than some parts of the world; but that does not prove that individually and collectively we treat everyone democratically. We cannot boast wholeheartedly that this is the land of opportunity and fair play until every child in the United States has a *real* opportunity to go through grade school, high school, junior college and beyond, *if his talents warrant it*. This would mean that the government would have to spend vastly more on education, including substantial scholarships for students, in order to prevent mere accidents of birth from being insuperable obstacles to advanced schooling. If one is born in a rural district, in a poor family, or of Negro parentage, the odds are heavily against his attending college or even the upper grades in some parts of the country. You may say, "Yes, but such a child has a *chance* if he really wants to get somewhere, for some very poor children by dint of great sacrifice, courage, and industry have risen to important places in the professional world and have even become famous." Only a few of the underprivileged, however, are blessed with such an indomitable spirit. The rest, who are not endowed with superhuman wills, are *practically* excluded from educational opportunities. Other children who have no greater native strength of character may secure a good education and enter a lucrative occupation simply because they were lucky enough to be born into the right family or the right community.

If these statements sound like exaggerations, they are none-the less true. School statistics prove them. In a rich state like California, for example, the illiteracy rate in 1930 was 2.6 per cent. In a poor state, South Carolina, the illiteracy rate was 14.9 per cent. Annual school expenditures per child in California in 1932 were $154.80, in South Carolina, $33.43. It will not add to our complacency to note that the birth rate in South Carolina has been approximately twice as high as the birth rate of California.

Racial Inequality

If we believe that life should be a race (with the slogan: May the best man or woman win!), an elementary sense of justice forces us to admit that it should be a fair race, with no one having a head start or suffering any handicap in so far as it is in our power to prevent injustices. Probably the most deep-seated kind of unfairness is racial prejudice. Our country has the unenviable distinction of being second only to India and a few other places in the cruel practice of making outcasts of millions of our citizens. There are historical reasons to account in part for our treatment of the Negro. Negroes were imported as slaves at a time when slavery was still almost universal. After the Civil War the unwise and high-handed policies of the northern carpet-baggers in prematurely setting up the Negroes in positions of political authority, caused much bitterness among southern whites, fear and hatred of the Negroes, and the establishment of lynch-law. At the present time, however, discrimination according to color is not a mere hang-over of the past. It is perpetuated by the fierce struggle for a livelihood and for preferred residential, medical, and recreational facilities. If we ever learn to control economic forces so that there will be a good-paying job for everyone who wants it, the chief cause of most racial antagonisms now existing among the lower income groups will be removed. In the meantime, Negroes come to bat with two strikes against them.

Incomes of Negroes and Whites. In 1935–36 Negro and white

incomes were compared by the National Resources Committee. It was discovered that in the rural South 80 per cent of the Negro families had incomes of less than $750 per year, whereas only 30 per cent of the white families failed to receive at least $750.* Every study of income distribution shows the same thing, viz., the Negro is at the bottom economically. There is dispute as to some of the reasons for this fact, but the outstanding cause is the exclusion of the Negro from the more skilled types of work. Farm labor, unskilled industrial labor, domestic service: these are the lowest rungs of the economic ladder. On these lowest rungs we find most of the Negroes who are gainfully employed. To take a city which is far from the extremes, viz., Chicago, we learn that in 1920 two-thirds of the working Negroes (male) were domestics or unskilled laborers. Less than one-third of the white employees were in those categories. Less than 7 per cent of the Negroes in Chicago were in the professions, in business or in public service.†

Medical Care for Negroes and Whites. The Julius Rosenwald Fund reported in 1942 some related evidences of discrimination. The tuberculosis death rate for Negroes was 129 per 100,000, three times the rate for the United States as a whole. The death rate (all causes) for Negroes was 14 per thousand, 32 per cent higher than for the country as a whole. There were only 10,000 hospital beds for 13,000,000 Negroes, and the entire South employed only 341 Negro public health nurses.

Educational opportunity, choice of occupation, and medical care are not the only privileges which tend to be granted and withheld according to class rather than according to strictly individual need or merit in the United States. Nor are Negroes and those who are born into poverty-stricken families the only persons who suffer from class distinctions. We have mentioned only the extreme cases. In every community there are many inequalities in rights, and discrimination in the treatment of human beings is made on the basis of many classifications besides ability and virtue.

America has never pretended to be a classless society. Some

* See "Consumer Incomes in the United States," report of the National Resources Committee, Sept. 4, 1938. Government Printing Office.
† E. Franklin Frazier, "Occupational Classes Among Negroes in Cities." *American Journal of Sociology*, 25:718–738, 1930.

inequalities are quite generally accepted, notably differences in income which recognize differences in the value and quantity of a person's work. Other inequalities are partially accepted, such as those based upon age and sex. But we may well give some thought to those inequalities that are justified by nothing except ancestry, the occupation or wealth of one's ancestors, facial appearance, and place of birth or residence. Especially when such accidents become the reason for extreme discrimination, they cannot be defended honestly, and the unrest of the underprivileged is a constant menace to the public peace and order. If we do not want strikes, riots, and sabotage, we should try to reduce these injustices. If we want the kind of efficiency that comes only from genuine cooperation, we should not support injustices.

Social Equality

If society maintained no irrational and undeserved class distinctions, we should still want to honor and reward those whose life and work were of especially great value to their fellows. But we should not want to reward the heroes and the geniuses by debasing ordinary folks. Even less should we do this in our present social system, where so·many honors and privileges are fortuitous.

Now one of the ways in which we can treat people democratically in spite of differences in achievement and reward is to cultivate the sense of social equality. This is a phase of democracy which has been developing slowly for centuries but has been intensified by the spirit of American frontier life. It would seem that most of the prejudice against social equality lies in the interpretation that it means: I must associate with any and everyone. When it is pointed out that one is under no compulsion to associate with all white people, yet one does not deny them social equality, and in the same way one would be under no compulsion to associate with all—or any for that matter—of the colored in offering them social equality, the prejudice vanishes. It is then seen that social equality means freedom to associate with anyone with whom you wish to associate—you to be the judge of the congeniality. The right to equal education and equal opportunity in business and professions then takes on a quite different hue. Let us see, there-fore, just what is involved in this personal, spiritual side of democracy.

The Value of Social Equality. Sometimes the greatest values of our lives are things, like the air we breathe, that we are least conscious of. Such a value is the American tradition of social democracy—the least tangible but most precious part of our democratic heritage. Other phases of democracy are easy to talk about, to see in operation, and to evaluate. But social democracy has almost a mystical quality. It is something that is not so much understood as vaguely felt. It cannot be described in terms of laws, such as those that insure the prime essentials of equality before the courts and at the polls. And it is of all forms of equality valued most as an end in itself and not as a means. We either like a democratic atmosphere and the *mores* of an equalitarian society or we don't, and few of us ever ask or care what the precise consequences of such a way of life may be. That there *are* important consequences is undoubtedly a fact and that social equality provides the strongest guarantee for other forms of equality may well be true. But we are usually so much preoccupied with social democracy as an end that we do not feel the need of evaluating it as a means. The true demo-crat values social equality so much for its own sake that, if he has it, he can cheerfully endure the loss of much else, and con-versely no society without it would be tolerable to him, how-ever rich and efficient and just it might be in other respects.

Newspapers once carried the story of an Italian, Frank Rusoti, a worker in a paper mill at Kalamazoo, Michigan, who re-nounced an Italian fortune rather than give up his American citizenship. His father, a wealthy civil engineer, left his estate to Rusoti, provided that he agree to live in Italy the rest of his life. Rusoti in refusing the inheritance said, "I would rather be a mill worker here than king of Italy. My American citizenship means more to me than any other possession."

Social democracy is intangible but real. It is based upon some-thing very deeply rooted in human nature, and that is the desire of everybody to *be* somebody. In its least subtle form this desire means that everybody enjoys applause, likes to have other people look up to him, likes to be appreciated. In its crude, unsublimated form this desire for social status may be a desire to subordinate someone else. My superiority is obtained through his inferiority, my being somebody means his being nobody, or at least not much of a body.

For those who do not like to see superiority achieved at the expense of others, the problem of morality and of democratic civilization becomes paradoxically: how can *everybody* be somebody? How can everybody be superior? Absurd as such universal superiority may appear, it is actually found among true friends. True friends constitute a sort of mutual admiration society in which everybody looks up to everybody else. This mutual respect, which is so essential to the highest type of friendship, is the basis of social democracy. It amounts to a guarantee of sufficient social status to all men so as to take the edge off of any differences which may occur above this minimum level of mutual esteem. Social democracy is thus a kind of feeling tone of *being somebody*, a sense of intrinsic dignity, which a democratic society undertakes to foster and defend in every citizen. It enables a person to admit that in reference to any specific human value—intelligence, good looks, athletic ability, wealth, fame, social grace—he may fall short, yet in his innermost self he knows that he is second to none. There is an essential soundness, validity, and worth about his personality, something that makes him feel the equal of the greatest and demand respect from the greatest, something that would prevent him from ever groveling before anyone, kow-towing to anyone, or accepting any class or caste as his "betters."*

With this sense of essential equality dominating his life, a person can be generous in granting superiority to other persons in any specific respect. He has a substantial, mystical, inner sort of dignity as his birthright. This is really what we mean when we say that "all men are created equal." We do not mean, any more than Thomas Jefferson meant, that all human beings will make the same scores on examinations or turn out the same amount of work in a day. Rather this chief tenet in the democratic creed affirms that there is something in the nature of man

* The Gallup Poll in 1939 revealed that only 6 per cent of the American people considered themselves among the lower class. 88 per cent called themselves "middle class" and 6 per cent "upper class."

as man which is worthy of respect. It refuses to see anyone suffer the ignominy of personal disrespect.

Surely, you will say, nurses do not have to be lectured on this subject. Of all professions nurses have the most humane attitude toward humanity. Yes, but . . . there are difficulties. Nurses can expect to deal with all kinds of people under every conceivable circumstance. It is not always easy to show just that considerateness of others which lets them know that they are not regarded as worthless. Let us consider two typical difficulties: (1) how to be democratic in an undemocratic institution, and (2) how to maintain professional relations with people who may take advantage of friendliness.

Being Democratic in an Undemocratic Institution

It would be easy to be democratic in a completely democratic world. The believer in equality, however, is confronted by a world that is democratic only in spots. A nurse, for example, may find that the hospital for which she works is one of the 1,577 hospitals* (out of 6,300 in the United States) that do not accept Negro patients. Or, perhaps, the hospital discriminates against Jews or members of some other religion. Or, she may be employed in a clinic where it is traditional to make poor people conscious of their poverty. Or, if, as is fortunately often the case, the medical institution is staffed by tolerant people, the outside community may be so prejudiced that doctors and nurses are suspected if they do not keep some minority group "in its place."

What complicates good intentions in such a situation is the fact that hospitals, clinics, and public health departments are usually in a precarious financial state. They are dependent upon the local community for patronage and support. Hence, a defiance of local prejudices may entail the wrecking of a much-needed medical program. To give certain patients the same class of service or to render service with the same cordiality that is accorded the elite may bring down the wrath of the "better element" either en masse or in the person of some "important

---

* According to a questionnaire survey of the American Medical Association in 1940.

person." Wrath may express itself in a boycott or the canceling of subscriptions or a demand for someone's job.

The course of wisdom cannot be prescribed *in general*. The democratic nurse, like the democratic doctor, will have to make an intelligent appraisal of the situation and decide which course of action will have the happiest or the least unhappy consequences. One general observation can, nevertheless, be advanced. There are many institutions which hold to undemocratic traditions not because of the power of undemocratic people but because of the *timidity* of democratic people. Faced with the kind of dilemma which we have just described, many persons of good intentions do nothing, and they try nothing. This is not as common in the field of health as it is in business and industry, but it is still very common for men and women to imagine formidable reactions to sensible reforms long after the opposition has become indifferent or powerless. "Nothing venture, nothing have." In saying this, we do not deny that there *are* American communities that are so undemocratic and unchristian that they are still pretty sure to punish tolerant and friendly people.

Institutions sometimes show disrespect for staff members as well as for members of their clientele. Although the beginner and the subordinate sometimes cry "Tyranny!" when there has been only a necessary exercise of authority, the fact remains that there are genuine tyrants in the United States. The Scientific Management engineers have distinguished the rational manager from the "temperamental" manager. The latter runs things by showing who is boss and by showing off. Discipline is maintained by making a subordinate "feel like a worm." Suggestions are not welcome. The reason for orders is never explained. And, perhaps, fawning is rewarded.

A nurse who finds herself in a tyrannized institution may not only resent the treatment which she receives, but if she has a supervisory position she may have a difficult time deciding how she will treat her subordinates. Again, a utilitarian has to say that each predicament of this sort will have to be judged according to its own merits. It may be that professional opportunities are so great that dictatorship can temporarily be endured. It may be that the tyrant is not as tyrannical as the first impression suggested. Quite possibly, the nurse will have to give thanks that this is a free country and seek other employment. Or, by sticking it out the nurse may help to usher in a more democratic regime. Especially in the last case, the first principle of organizational work needs to be remembered, viz., that the right to formulate rules and policies usually has to be earned. However bright the novice's ideas, the novice has to "work into the organization." Whether it be a hospital, a public health department, a school, a political party, or a club, large organizations nearly always require a period of apprenticeship before they are ready to respond to an individual's proposals. A democrat, like anyone else who aspires to influence in an institution, must have the patience of a democrat. But this counsel of patience has to do only with the means of securing genuine respect for human personality. Social equality remains as the goal, and one should be ready for the moment when a firm stand will result in the democratization of an institution.

Being Democratic AND Professional

The second difficulty with being democratic is that a friendly attitude is sometimes misinterpreted. There are individuals who are used to being treated "like a dog," and if anyone shows them any respect or amiability, they may try to take advantage of what they mistake for egregious good nature. A nurse may be tempted to appear "hard as nails" just so that she will not be imposed upon. There are also a few physicians and fellow-nurses who, unfortunately, are looking for an easy mark. The same may be said of a few clergymen, lawyers, social workers, military men, and representatives of other professions with whom nurses occasionally have to work. Certainly in dealing with patients and the relatives of patients, almost every experienced nurse has encountered the individual who, as soon as he detects any good will, assumes that the nurse is ready to forget her professional duty. Requests are made for ignoring the doctor's orders, for violating institutional rules, for special favors, for overtime and unreasonable extras, for ignoring the patient's welfare, for undue familiarity, etc.

Here, too, the difficulty is that we live in a world that is only partially democratic. Part of the offenders are underprivileged people who are so used to unkindness and injustice that they are incapable of the friendship of equals. The others are predatory and uncivilized. From our experiences with them we should learn something about democracy and good will. In order to harbor and manifest a fundamental good will towards human beings, it is not necessary to embrace them. "The brotherhood of man" cannot be the unlimited affection which we give to our family and our intimate friends. As Aristotle pointed out, affection simply will not spread that far. And, as we have seen, it is unwise. Yet, for all the reserve which is necessary in our dealings with some people, and despite the importance of preserving our professional standing in our professional relationships, it is still possible to serve most human beings without that condescension which says, "You are a nobody." In most American institutions it is possible to maintain discipline without exercising authority in a way that says, "You have no value." Where smiles and pleasantries are apt to be misinterpreted, the believer in democratic equality can manifest respect for human dignity at least by listening to the other person's point of view and by offering intelligible explanations of one's own actions and decisions.

To sum up: a person who has a fundamental respect for the personality of other human beings cannot be entirely satisfied as long as any of these human beings are denied decent opportunities because of the accident of birth or ancestry. But, however limited may be the democrat's power to correct present injustices, the democrat can express his desire to maintain social equality in day-to-day conduct in many different ways.

Study Questions

1. Name the nine rights that were defined by the National Resources Planning Board.
2. What handicaps and discriminations must be removed before complete equality of opportunity will be attained in this country?
3. What are the chief causes of racial discrimination? How can we reduce racial discrimination?
4. What do we really mean when we say that all men are

created free and equal or when we say that in a democracy one person is just as good as another?

5. Is there a conflict between the duty of maintaining professional status and the duty to be friendly?
6. What are the dangers in the expression of good will to patients? to subordinates? to tradesmen? to employers?
7. What are some of the problems of being democratic while working in an undemocratic institution?
8. Does the ideal of social equality require that everyone should receive the same enjoyments?

Questions for Thought and Discussion

1. What is the extent of racial discrimination in your community? How far can hospitals go toward the elimination of discrimination without suffering loss of support or patronage?
2. In certain states colored graduate nurses are not admitted to membership in the state nurses' association; they are, therefore, barred from membership in the American Nurses' Association. Do you think that the A.N.A. should admit colored nurses to individual membership? What would be the advantages and disadvantages?
3. Does the National Association of Colored Graduate Nurses offer sufficient opportunity for cooperative professional activity for colored nurses?
4. Give examples of the failure to attain the ideal of social equality.
5. Give examples of famous Americans who emerged from poverty. Do you think that the chances for rising out of a poor background are increasing or diminishing?
6. List the privileges of upper class membership.
7. List the bases of class distinction. Check your observations by consulting John Dollard's *Caste and Class in a Southern Town*. (Yale University Press, 1937) or E. S. Bogardus, *Immigration and Race Attitudes*. (D. C. Heath & Co., 1928) or H. W. Zorbaugh, *The Gold Coast and the Slum*. (University of Chicago Press, 1929.)

Books to Read

Smith, T. V.: *The Democratic Way of Life*, rev. ed. Chicago. University of Chicago Press. 1939.

Chase, Stuart: *Goals for America*. New York. The Twentieth Century Fund. 1942.

Leys, Wayne A. R.: *Ethics and Social Policy*. New York. Prentice Hall, Inc. 1941.

Committee on the Costs of Medical Care: *Medical Care for the American People*. Chicago. University of Chicago Press. 1932.

Bureau of Medical Economics, American Medical Association: *Handbook of Sickness Insurance, State Medicine and the Cost of Medical Care*. Chicago. American Medical Association Press. 1934.

XVI

Democratic Ideals

Throughout the discussion of nursing practices we have been aware of limitations which are imposed upon our good will by general social conditions. How often we have said in effect: "This is desirable, but we have to be practical." Plato and Aristotle seem to have been correct in their opinion that an individual can behave perfectly only in a perfect society. When we consider the questions of racial and class discriminations, when we face the problems of marriage and a career, when we examine the duties of a nurse, we are, in almost every case, confronted by certain barriers which we as individuals cannot completely surmount. We live in a world of warring groups, of poverty, and of irrationality. In fact, the existence of these impediments is the underlying reason for preferring an experimental, utilitarian ethics to a morality of absolute rules. Unable to predict the conditions which will arise from year to year and from place to place we must be prepared to evaluate conduct according to its variable consequences. Action which would have the happiest consequences in one situation may result in misery in the next.

Nurses are not the only specialists who have to adjust their policies to practical considerations. Engineers, teachers, physicians, artists, social workers, merchandisers—they are all restrained in the improvement of their respective services by general social conditions.

All of us, therefore, have the problem of orienting ourselves and getting our bearings in the larger scene so as to see more clearly what we can do. Shall we look upon the fundamental structure of society with the same resignation with which we view the weather? Or shall we recognize in the complex problems, which no single professional group can solve, a need and

an opportunity for the collaboration of all occupational groups?
A believer in democracy will prefer to look upon the fundamental ills of society as common problems demanding the joint
efforts of all classes and all specialists.

In the twentieth century the great common problems of
achieving peace, health, liberty, and justice all have an economic
aspect. They are also political problems, but we shall grapple
with poverty and unemployment in the hope that such economic
facts will reveal the nature of our most pervasive difficulties.

Economic Inequality

Before the war, when we were just coming out of the depression, some studies of actual family budgets were made for the
U. S. Department of Labor. One class of family studied averaged
a little over $2 per week for food per member and paid about
$20 a month rent. Was this the average American family or
was it below average? As a matter of fact it was above average.
Its annual income was $1,500 while the median family's income
was only $1,160. Three-fifths of all families had a *worse* living
than did this one.

In order to appreciate more fully the sort of living which this
better-than-average family had, let us look at their entire
budget:*

Food	$555	Amusement	$30
Clothing	120	Tobacco	30
Housing & Household Operation	450	Reading	15
Furniture	30	Education	7
Automobile or Transportation	85	Direct taxes, gifts, etc	28
Personal Care	30	Insurance	60
Medical and Dental Care	60	Total	$1,500

If this family had about five members and lived in a city, we
can well imagine in what sort of house and in what an inferior
neighborhood it lived and how meager was its living all around.
A thoughtful analysis of each item will reveal the details of the
family's life. What sort of car could be owned and operated on
$85 a year minus other kinds of transportation costs? What
sort of medical and dental care could be obtained for five persons
on an average of $60 a year? Assuming that half the amusement

* Based on Bulletin 5626 of U. S. Department of Labor, Jan. 2, 1938.

allowance went for movies, how many movies could a family of five see on a little over a dollar a month? How much life and health insurance could be obtained for $60 a year? Or if savings took the place of insurance, how much could such a family save for old age in thirty years?

The Average Family. We ordinarily imagine the average American family as enjoying a pretty comfortable living—a nice house in a good neighborhood, good, wholesome food without much skimping, neat-looking clothes, a pretty good car, all the medical and dental attention they need, frequent attendance at movies, and other similar items. This was certainly an illusion even in 1936 when we had recovered from the depression somewhat. The median family with an income of $1,160 could not have dreamed of such "luxuries." And as for families in the lowest third, President Roosevelt was right in describing them as ill-housed, ill-clothed, and ill-fed.

Let us see just how the national income was distributed among some 29,400,300 families (comprising 91 per cent of the population) in the fiscal year 1935–36:*

Distribution of National Income, 1935–1936

	FAMILIES		AGGREGATE INCOME		
Income Level	Percentage of Families	Cumulative Percentage	Income in Millions of Dollars	Percentage of Total Income	Cumulative Percentage
0– 999.....	41.68	41.68	7,424	15.57	15.57
1,000– 1,499.....	22.95	64.63	8,256	17.32	32.89
1,500– 1,999.....	14.42	79.05	7,246	15.19	48.08
2,000– 2,499.....	8.38	87.43	5,474	11.48	59.56
2,500– 2,999.....	4.47	91.90	3,569	7.48	67.04
3,000– 4,999.....	5.39	97.29	5,780	12.12	79.16
5,000– 9,999.....	1.74	99.03	3,506	7.36	86.52
10,000–19,999.....	.65	99.68	2,510	5.27	91.79
20,000–49,999.....	.27	99.95	2,265	4.76	96.55
50,000–99,999.....	.04	99.99	755	1.58	98.13
100,000– and over...	.01	100.	894	1.87	100.

What significance do these figures have for us today? They indicate the condition we were in before the boom of war

* *Consumer Incomes in the United States, July 1, 1935–July 1, 1936, National Resources Committee, August, 1938.*

employment came. The income of all persons in the United States in 1936 amounted to around 60 billion dollars. There were possibly 12 million unemployed. With full employment we might have had a national income of ninety billion dollars or more on the basis of prices existing at that time. Congress did not take the steps necessary to put everyone to work. The ordinary, every-day insecurity and poverty of millions of people was not felt to be a national emergency, and only the threat of outright starvation of large numbers could bring action. Congress did only enough to keep the number of unemployed from reaching dangerous proportions. As for guaranteeing to every person a good, respectable job as his birth-right, very few politicians felt this to be a political obligation. Congressmen and newspapers and most of the public spent more time deploring the large national debt than worrying about the huge waste of idle man-power and the destruction of human morale and happiness.

Solution of Unemployment Problem during War. But when the nation was attacked, that was an emergency which everyone could visualize. All of our instincts of self-preservation, as well as our hatred of undemocratic, ruthless peoples, impelled us to go all out to win the war. We were willing to do *anything* to achieve victory. The sky was the limit as far as the national debt was concerned, and no one obstructed the war effort by asking how we were ever going to pay it back. The result was that we were able to put almost all of our unemployed to work. Indeed, if we had not had to expend half of our energy on war-production, we could have enjoyed the highest level of living we had ever known.

This comparison between what we failed to do during the depression and what we showed ourselves we could do, when we made up our minds to do it, during the war, has taught us a lesson. We know that if we *want* to find ways of employing everyone we can do it. Also, the fact that dictatorships have been able to solve the unemployment problem has become a challenge to our democracy. We do not care to use their methods, of course, but we know that we must find democratic methods to achieve the same results.

Employment and Purchasing Power

In the opinion of some economists, our problem under capitalism is to attain full employment by increasing the purchasing
power of the nation to the limit of our productive capacity, and
then to stabilize, i.e., to see to it that expenditures never decline.
In the past, they say, we depended upon the natural growth of
the country, the rapid expansion of factories, and new inventions to cause business men to borrow money to be used to
create capital goods and indirectly to employ men and increase
purchasing power all around. But our pioneering days are over,
our population is no longer increasing rapidly, industry is not
being revolutionized every few years as it once was; rather
changes in methods of production are gradual and continuous
and do not require vast new outlays of capital. It is necessary,
therefore, for the federal government henceforth to take the
responsibility of stimulating our economic system so as to
create and maintain the greatest possible purchasing power and
employment. This has to be done first by borrowing and spending and secondly by controlling the distribution of incomes
through taxation so that the nation's income as a whole will
be spent as rapidly as it is earned.

Ideas of Personal Economy Not Applicable to Nation as a Whole.
In order that we may support the government in such a program
—so runs the argument—we must rid ourselves of certain
habits of thought. We all agree that for *individuals* it is bad to
borrow money unless absolutely necessary; secondly, we are
placing a burden upon our future when we do borrow; and,
thirdly, we must certainly intend to pay our debts back as soon
as possible. But none of these rules apply to the *nation as a whole.*
A large national debt does no harm, but good, if we can stimu-
late employment by it. It does not put a burden upon the nation
as a whole in the future because the money that the government
pays in interest charges is not lost but is received by American
citizens and can be used to purchase goods and services. It is
true that someone has to pay taxes to enable the government
to pay interest but this means then that maintaining the debt
just results in a redistribution of incomes. We rob Peter to pay
Paul but the total level of living of the nation remains just as
high as it would be if there were no debt. And, if those are

taxed most heavily who have excess income, the redistribution of incomes may be a positive good. Finally, it is not necessary to pay the debt back, since the government can always issue new bonds to pay off old ones and, as long as the interest charges can be met through taxation, the existence of the debt does no harm. In fact, if the government launched out on a program of curtailing expenses in order to pay off the debt, this would just mean unemployment and another depression.

We are also told that another rule of conduct which is desirable for individuals but not for the federal government is economy. This does not mean that the government should be wasteful of resources and labor but it means that we should stop complaining when the government spends millions or even billions of dollars. Government borrowing, government spending, and the resulting increased taxes are good things if they result in full employment and a better living for most of the nation, and equal opportunity for all. If it is feared that there will not be enough useful work on which the government may spend its money, just consider how badly the nation needs (a) better housing, (b) more medical services, (c) more education, and (d) conservation of resources, and all fears of "boondoggling" will disappear.

An even more tradition-smashing view concerns taxes; namely, that we must get away from our habit of regarding taxation as an evil. The old phrase "as certain as death and taxes" places taxes next to the greatest evil of human existence. But modern taxation respresents much more than keeping up expensive government bureaus. It may be used as a beneficent instrument to make the capitalistic system work by redistributing incomes and increasing or maintaining purchasing power.

To contrast once more individual ethics and wise national policy, it is desirable for most individuals to spend less than they earn and put away savings for a future emergency or old age, but it would be disastrous for the whole nation to spend less than it earns. In order to maintain the same amount of employment and the same national income from year to year it is necessary for the nation as a whole to spend the same amount of money each year. Since spending less than has been earned in the previous year would mean throwing people out of work, the business of the government is to watch to see whether some classes of people are making so much that they cannot spend it or invest it in new securities, and, if this is the case, it is necessary to take their excess savings away from them by taxation for the good of the country.

What would this policy achieve? Its proponents claim that it would maintain employment at any existing level. Naturally we should not be content with anything less than full employment with the highest level of national income possible. If, they say, we are at any point below this, the function of the government becomes not merely to stabilize at a given level but to raise the level by seeing to it that the nation spends more than it makes every year until maximum employment is reached. This may be done either by encouraging the expansion of credit, or borrowing by private business, or through government borrowing and spending.

Expansion of Purchasing Power and Price Control. Danger points in the plan have been seen and provided for. In a program of expansion, one thing that has to be watched is the possibility that rises in prices may cancel out all the increases in purchasing power which are being created. Hence the government may have to continue to set ceilings for prices in peace as well as in war. It is very foolish for business men to raise prices when they learn that the public is going to have more money to spend. An individual is likely to think that he might as well cash in on a little extra profit by raising prices a bit, but if everybody does this the public has no more money to spend relative to prices asked than it had before, and the demand for real goods is no greater and employment is not increased at all. So by such short-sighted greed, we kill the goose that might lay the golden eggs. Unless we have reached the limit of our resources and there is a scarcity of goods, it is logical for prices to be reduced rather than increased when the demand increases, for with a larger volume of business, overhead costs are usually less per unit of production and call for a lowering of prices. At any rate, if business men are not wise enough to see this, then the government will have to prohibit price rises when it is attempting to increase employment.

Would such government power imply "dictatorship"? Those who believe in the plan say not. They consider that the methods by which the change is brought about make all the difference. In this country these methods could be humane and democratic instead of inhuman and arbitrary as in dictatorships.

Conclusion: There are many difficulties—political and economic—connected with the program outlined above or indeed with any program offered us today. We are not able here to elaborate upon these. We may conclude, however, by stressing the fact that the future of capitalism in this country will depend upon whether we solve the unemployment problem by measures other than war. The people have at last become conscious of their right to work, and no economic system and no government in the future can long endure without meeting this demand.

International Inequality

International economics present much the same picture as national economics: unemployment and over-production occurring simultaneously. War came in 1939 in part because of the inability of the most powerful nations to work out a satisfactory arrangement for the exchange of raw materials and finished goods. In the absence of such trade agreements the factories of industrial countries were idle while the non-industrial nations suffered for want of the goods which these factories could have supplied.

We are all familiar with the phrase "the haves and the have-nots." The Nazi propagandists completely misrepresented the international inequalities, but that should not blind us to the existence of such inequalities. Germany and Japan were not the real have-nots. Poland and China were among the real have-nots; their standards of living were far below the income levels of their invaders. Germany and Japan were not the richest nations, but that was not their real reason for aggression.

To understand the international situation it is necessary to look at an industrial map of the world in the period between the great wars. If industrial regions are marked in red and non-industrial regions are colored green, most of the earth's land surface will be green. The factory system is an application of scientific discoveries and inventions, and the application has not been universal. First, northern England and then the northwest corner of the European continent developed the industrial arts. Somewhat later textile mills, steel mills, etc. appeared in the northeastern part of the United States. Still later came the industrialization of Japan, Russia, and scattered localities in Australia, India, etc. This was the extent of industrialization in the late twenties and early thirties.

The rest of the world was not, however, unaffected. South America, the southern and western parts of the United States, southeastern Europe, Africa, Manchuria, etc. were at the same time being transformed economically. Instead of remaining with a self-sufficient agriculture these "backward regions" were converting to mining and export agriculture. In other words, the backward regions were supplying raw materials to the industrial centers and they were buying part of the finished goods.

Decline of International Trade. Conceivably, this kind of imperialistic trade could have been profitable and satisfactory to all concerned. But such was not the case. Because of superior bargaining power the industrial centers made very large profits on their colonial trade. (Within the United States the northeastern industries made large profits on their trade with the west and the south.) For a time this large profit was quite useful because it enabled the industries of the world to build up their capital equipment: plants, machines, transportation systems, etc. Eventually this large profit margin disrupted international trade. "Backward countries" began to build factories in order to reap the benefits of industrialism. This caused a scramble for markets and for sources of raw materials. In order not to reduce prices and their profit margins a number of industrial countries, especially in central Europe, tried to protect their home markets by high tariffs and to grab new markets by an amazing variety of means. The trouble was that every country could do the same. The economic warfare of the late twenties and early thirties consisted of a vicious circle of retaliatory tariffs and currency manipulations. The result was a virtual cessation of world trade. International trade had amounted to 68 billion dollars in 1929. In 1932 it had slumped to 24 billion dollars.

So it was that factories were idle in the industrial countries, and in the non-industrial regions mines were idle while the prices of agricultural products fell to ruinously low levels. This gave the militarists in Japan, Germany, and Italy their opportunity. They appealed to the unemployed (capitalists as well as workingmen), and put men and machines back to work—making armaments.

Once a war is in the making, all kinds of objectives get associated with the military enterprise. We can see, however, what the long-range strategy of the German militarists was in the late thirties. They hoped to do the manufacturing, if not for the whole world, then for Europe, Africa, and South America. In a word, they wished to concentrate industry even more than before, dismantling factories in other European countries and moving them to the Reich. Then, with all of their neighbors reduced to the disadvantageous position of raw-material regions, the Germans would accumulate the profits and live high.

In the anti-Axis governments, particularly in 1939, there were a good many people who saw nothing wrong with an unbalanced imperialist economy. They may not have wanted to concentrate manufacturing further, but they were well satisfied with an industrial-colonial trade, provided that other industrial nations did not encroach upon their markets and sources of supply.

Internationalism Vs. Isolationism. As for the democratic people who did not want an economic imperialism, they were divided into two camps: the extreme isolationists* and the internationalists. The extreme isolationists were prepared to stop all international trading. When they were in control of the American Congress, they passed the Neutrality Acts, which called for prohibition of all travel by Americans in war zones, so that no incident of an American life lost in a war zone could be made an incident to draw us into war (as sinking of the Lusitania was used in World War I); of sale of munitions to any belligerent country; and of sale of any non-war products unless moved in

---

* We must distinguish the extreme isolationists from the pseudo-isolationists. The latter do not wish their government to make any international commitments but at the same time they wish to extend their country's trade in all parts of the world. Thus, they would have the profits of international trade but dodge any responsibility for keeping that trade peaceful and orderly.

ships not flying the United States flag (cash and carry). That these last two would reduce the American standard of living, some of the extreme isolationists were ready to admit; but they preferred a lower standard of living to entanglement in international conflicts.

The trend of events proved that extreme isolation is impossible in a world of rapid transportation. Did it prove that the internationalists had a vision of the way out? The internationlists saw the trouble as arising, at least in part, from the unbalanced world economy. Because of unequal bargaining power, profits from international trade were greater in the industrial regions than in the mining and agricultural regions. After the manufacturing countries had accumulated a certain amount of capital, they should have reduced their prices for finished goods and thus increased the purchasing power of their own laboring classes as well as the purchasing power of the "backward" peoples. Putting the matter another way, the internationalist contended that the time had come to devote more work and capital to the production of things that consumers use and less work and capital to the production of machines and factories. Yet, in every manufacturing region the distribution of income was such that profits continued to pile up and the recipients of the profits tried to invest in profitable enterprises. At a time when the United States had more factories than were needed to make all of the shoes and cotton cloth that consumers could buy, investors continued to put their profits into the construction of more shoe factories and textile mills.

The internationalist whose views are affected by idealism as well as economics believes that sooner or later the world's income must be redistributed so that more will go to the people who would increase their consumption of shoes, clothing, food, etc. and less will go to the people who now have incomes far in excess of their consumption needs and who therefore try to build more and more factories. This redistribution may be effected in many ways, and it would be foolish to say that just one method should be employed. The prices of manufactured goods could be lowered. Wages could be raised. Surplus profits could be taxed and used by the governments to improve public services. Tariffs could be lowered. Or, as occurred to some extent in the Lend-Lease administration during the war, there could be direct gifts to other countries.

The intricacies of international economics are too complex to explain fully in a brief discussion. The only point which we wish to emphasize in this section is that the bugaboo of international industry is the same as the bugaboo of domestic industry: unequal bargaining power gives some parties such excessive profits that they presently have more factories and more transportation facilities than can be kept busy. Unless a slave-system, such as the Nazis visualized, is set up, the more powerful and the more fortunate must lose some of their pursuit of profits for themselves and help to raise the standard of living of the rest of the world.

> "In the past, the typical industrial enterprise has had one main purpose—profits—and the industrial system as a whole, in the view of liberals, has had another—multiplying products for consumers. The theory, as already pointed out, was that competition led producers to promote the second while aiming at the first; and at times the practice agreed to a fair extent with the theory. Adequate employment is a different sort of objective; and at present we do not seem likely to find a magic formula whereby industry will promote this objective in spite of itself, while aiming primarily at something else. It seems to be the kind of thing industry must aim at consciously and directly if the system is to promote it."[*]

The Right to Health

When the economist talks about the problem of distribution, he is using his own language to discuss the problem of applying modern science. Engineers, chemists, and other specialists have solved the problems of production:, they know how certain goods can be made and how they can be transported. The baffling question is how to make these goods available to the people who could use them without inviting quarrels, laziness, and waste.

[*] J. M. Clark, "The Democratic Concept in the Economic Realm." *Science, Philosophy, and Religion: Third Symposium,* p. 179. Conference on Science, Philosophy and Religion, 1943.

If the general problem of distribution sounds academic to some nurses (as it does to many others), perhaps we should see how it presents itself in connection with medical science. On the evidence of vital statistics we should say that the people of the United States enjoy much better medical care than the average. Our life expectancy (more than 60 years) is double that of Latin America. In South and Central America, except for Uruguay and Argentina, tuberculosis rates run as high as six times the U. S. rate. Yellow fever, smallpox, malaria, typhus and dysentery are so prevalent that at least fifty million of the one hundred twenty millions south of the Rio Grande are sick at the present moment.*

No, we have a much better record. Medical science knows how to control bubonic plague, and we have applied our science Medical science knows how to control smallpox, and we have applied our knowledge in most regions within the United States. Even the poor receive more scientific medical services than kings did a hundred years ago.

Failure to Utilize Medical Science. But, wait. Let us look at the health statistics again. There were 2,664 cases of diphtheria in Illinois during 1935. Is the prevention of diphtheria unknown? No, the immunization measures have been standardized, but they are not used everywhere. How does it happen that 13,221 persons died of syphilis in the United States in 1937? Was there no effective treatment? There was, but some infections were not detected soon enough. Why does New Mexico have an astounding infant mortality rate? Is the New Mexican climate particularly unhealthful? No, the answer is poverty and the lack of physicians and nurses in the sparsely settled districts. Is it beyond the power of science to maintain a better state of health than was revealed by the selective service rejections? Certainly not.

Science is still baffled by a few diseases, but a number of ailments that are still high on the mortality and prevalence tables were either preventable or curable years ago. The problem is to *distribute* medical skill and nursing care.

* Estimate of C. M. Wilson, "How Latin Americans Die and What We Can Do About It." *Harpers Magazine*, July, 1942, pp. 141–148.

The following statement by a member of a state board of health will make conditions more graphic:

> In this state approximately one-third of the people die without consulting a doctor even in their fatal illness. In six of its thirty-one counties, less than one quarter of the mothers have medical care in childbirth. In seven of this state's counties more than three-quarters of the babies that die have had no medical care. A conservative estimate from a health survey of this state made two years ago places the number of cases of active tuberculosis at not less than 15,000. At present there are no free beds for tuberculosis and very few of these patients can pay for sanatorium care. There is no provision for surgical treatment to save the patient's life and stop the spread of infection. The same survey proves that there are in the state 20,000 people whose blood shows the presence of syphilis. Only one thousand are under the care of a physician. The infant mortality in this state is the highest in the union. It was 126.1 per 1,000 live births in 1935.*

Other illuminating examples showing the inadequacy of medical care are the following: In two counties in Kentucky of 8,700 and 10,000 inhabitants, there was only one licensed physician in each, at the time the reports in *American Medicine* were written. Similar instances can be found in other states. In one county all indigent patients were handled by one physician whose salary was $1400 a year, out of which he had to pay about $200 for gas and oil and $365 for drugs and supplies. After these deductions were made his rate of services were computed to be about 8 cents per call at office, home, or hospital. Among other things, in one year he handled 55 obstetrical cases and did 5 hysterectomies, 72 other abdominal operations, 25 tonsillectomies, 11 operations for hemorrhoids, 3 eye operations, 2 cancer operations, 1 gallbladder operation and a number of other miscellaneous operations, not to mention extracting 542 teeth.†

* *American Medicine*, Vol. I, page 20. Published by The American Foundation, 565 Fifth Ave., New York, 1937.
† *American Medicine*, Vol. II, page 1187.

Health for Everyone—Its Cost. This must suffice to show what a stupendous task confronts us in providing health for everyone. To attain our goal is going to take a great deal of education of ourselves and others. And it is going to cost money. At present according to a pamphlet of the Public Affairs Committee, the cost of all medical and dental services per capita is $30 a year.* The author of this pamphlet presents the estimate that for $36 per capita adequate provisions for health could be made for the entire population, if the services were most efficiently organized. If our conjecture as to the real medical needs of the country is at all correct, then this estimate of $36 is far too small. Double the present expenditure would probably be required to deliver the best type of health service to the entire nation. But even at $60 per capita we would be getting one of the greatest values in life for a trifling sum.

Can we afford to pay $60 per year for health? That would mean $300 per year for a family of five. Certainly there are many families which do not now spend $300 a year for medical and dental care who could spend that much without skimping on necessities or denying themselves a reasonable amount of luxuries. The difficulty with these middle income families is that their medical needs do not occur at regular intervals. Moreover, medical needs are not evenly distributed among families. Ten families may have virtually no ills for five years, and suddenly one of them will require services that cost $5,000. The physicians, the nurses, the pharmacist, and the hospital could be paid if the afflicted family had been saving for a rainy day or if the care-free families would help out the afflicted family. But, human nature being what it is, neither of these possibilities happens very often.

Health Insurance. To make sure that middle class families of limited means reserve enough income for the health service which they expect, a number of schemes have been devised: voluntary health insurance or pre-payment of medical and

* See *Doctors, Dollars, and Disease,* Public Affairs Pamphlet, No. 10, 1937, prepared by William I. Foster on the basis of the studies of the Committee on the Costs of Medical Care and reports of the American Hospital Association, the American College of Surgeons, the American Medical Association, and the United States Public Health Service. Published by the Public Affairs Committee, National Press Building, Washington, D. C. (10 cents).

hospital bills and compulsory health insurance. At present the most generally approved plan for the middle classes is that of hospital insurance. This idea originated at the Baylor University Hospital in 1929 and has now spread throughout the country until many millions of people are using it. The American Hospital Association aids communities in organizing hospitalization projects. The rates and provisions of this insurance vary, but as a rule a person receives for around ten dollars per year the right to occupy a semi-private room for as long as three weeks. He is entitled also to the use of ambulance, operating room and various laboratory services without extra charge. Obstetrical and other cases may be excluded or granted half rates.

Pre-payment of medical services commonly takes two forms. The first is an arrangement by which a certain sum of money is paid by an individual for himself or his family to a county medical society, or to a health insurance company,* which reimburses the family physician at a standard rate whenever medical services are required. The other scheme involves group practice. That is, a group of physicians practice cooperatively and guarantee all types of medical service to patients who pay a stipulated sum each year. This type of insurance has been tried out most extensively on the west coast.

There are many problematical features about both hospital insurance and medical pre-payment plans, and it should be recognized that in many cases they do not yet provide as complete services as would be ideal, for the rates are too low for this. We cannot expect to obtain ideal medical service for a mere song. But even rather limited medical services for certain employed groups constitute a great improvement over anything they have previously enjoyed.

Compulsory health insurance, while quite common for workers in Europe, is not looked upon with favor by many physicians in this country. It is generally feared that compulsory insurance would open the way for an unwholesome control of medicine by politicians and that, combined with free choice of physician, it would give an advantage to unethical physicians who might use

* Group Health Mutual, Inc., in St. Paul, Minnesota, has avoided conflict with the medical profession by having members pay their annual fees to Group Health Mutual and then the latter pays reasonable fees to physicians on the basis of services rendered to individual members.

various direct and indirect ways of advertising themselves. Certainly any scheme of compulsory health insurance which does not give a large measure of control in its administration to the medical profession itself is to be regarded with misgiving.

There is much to be said for the application of the insurance principle to health risks. Each of the aforementioned plans spreads medical and hospital costs over a period of time and over a number of families, so that the necessary part of income is available when the expenses are incurred.

The insurance type of financing, however, is totally inadequate for a large part of the population. The reason for this is fairly obvious. A family whose income is $1100 per year can scarcely set aside $300 or even $150 for medical expenses without skimping on food or rent or clothing. The situation is much worse for $750 and $900 families, of whom there are many in the rural regions.

At this point medical economics must be related to economics in general. The main problem is that of increasing the total income of great masses of people. As was suggested in the preceding section, there are several ways in which this can be done. If wages and employment are increased generally or if the prices of certain commodities are lowered, there would naturally be more money available for doctors, nurses, dentists, and hospitals. The insurance type of financing would then be possible for a larger proportion of the patients.

Socialized Medicine. In the absence of a permanent raising of purchasing power, another scheme for more adequate health service is state medicine, or socialized medicine, as it is often called. The government uses its taxing power to take surplus industrial profits and appropriates these funds for health work. On a small scale this has been done for a long period—in fact, ever since the establishment of public health departments. During the past fifteen years public health appropriations have increased, not only to pay for the care of paupers but also to subsidize hospitals and laboratories and health work in the public schools.

If America's medical budget is to be expanded by government financing rather than by a general increase in purchasing power, there are undoubtedly some dangers to be reckoned with. The chief hazard to be avoided is the control of hospitals and medical services by politicians instead of by the medical staff. Closely related is the danger that an attempt will be made to expand the health services without adequate appropriations.

It is easy to engage in a purely speculative argument about the pros and cons of state medicine. If the hospitals connected with state university medical schools are examined, some of them will be found to supply the finest medical service in the country. They are controlled by the medical staff rather than by politicians, and, although the doctors and nurses are on salaries, there is nothing communistic about the enterprise, since they do not all receive the same salary. The units are large enough so that the best known medical and surgical equipment can be provided at minimum cost.

The danger of ignorant political control depends to a large extent upon the vigilance of the experts and also upon the establishment of a system that is not too highly centralized. As Justice Brandeis contended, there are limits to the size of human organizations beyond which bureaucratic red tape is sure to appear. The problem is to develop the administrative arts and devise a workable plan for distributing health services in the United States.

However much disagreement there may be concerning the way to do it, the main objective is to guarantee the right to health to more human beings. We know that this necessitates the wider application of medical knowledge that is already accumulated, as well as progress in further research. To use more widely the discoveries of Pasteur and Osler and other geniuses we must have more physicians, more nurses, and more equipment. To support the physicians and nurses and to pay for the equipment we must make more income available for health purposes. We know that production, including the production of health services, can be increased. Our question is which of several alternative methods shall be used.

Political Equality

Some persons who see the possibilities of applying science for the benefit of more and more human beings are brought to despair when they encounter stupid and selfish opposition to the actual use of our knowledge. They look for no improvement unless through violent revolution and dictatorship. English-speaking peoples and others of long democratic traditions, on the other hand, believe that they can solve the economic problems in an orderly way without sacrificing the democratic privileges of free speech and press and popular elections. We believe that, in spite of temporary inefficiency, democratic societies will attain their goal of widespread happiness sooner than other kinds of government and with less sacrifice in the process. At least we are quite sure that this is true of ourselves, even though it may not have been true for countries that did not have a democratic tradition.

In order to make sure, however, that our congressmen and other representatives of the people are wise enough to steer our ship of state through the troubled waters of the post-war world, we need to inquire into the processes by which they are selected and controlled. In doing this we shall become conscious of some of the shortcomings of our political democracy and the need for removing these.

Participation in Politics. Theoretically, political democracy means basic equality of power among the people, or equal opportunity to control the government. For this, equal suffrage at the polls is, of course, essential. But of equal importance is active participation in party organizations by large numbers of citizens so that the nomination of candidates is not left in the hands of a small clique of professional politicians. Without equality of participation in politics, the mere right to vote is not sufficient.

Democracy has often been criticized on the ground that it tends to put mediocre persons into office rather than the best. As a matter of fact, in many of our city governments we have done worse than elect merely average men—we have elected men who were below average in honesty, if not in ability. In our national government we have done better, though we still fall far short of the ideal of electing the best men or women to represent us.

This is not due to the fact that the masses of people are naturally stupid and cannot recognize capable candidates. But it is the result of the failure of democracy to adapt itself to urban civilization. We are suffering from bigness—the fact that our relationships are impersonal and we no longer carry out our political functions in face-to-face contact with our neighbors. The break-down of democracy may be seen when we go to the polls and receive a ballot upon which we are supposed to indicate our choices from among some hundred names. We may not be able to recognize more than a half dozen candidates and of those we may have very little accurate information. And the fact that an intelligent person is as much at a loss to know how to vote as an unintelligent one is evidence that there is something wrong with the *system*.

Only in small communities where voters can come together in town meetings in which they are acquainted with most people present, and certainly with the candidates for office, can democracy be said to function fully. There, if poor officials are selected, it is clearly the fault of the people. As a matter of fact, however, the candidates selected in such meetings are usually well above the average. And if a mistake is made, everyone knows precisely how to correct it at the next session, whereas in large cities a majority of the citizens may know that there is much corruption and inefficiency in the government and not know where to turn to correct it. Democracy thus degenerates when most voters feel that they have lost touch with their government and can only stand on the sidelines and "gripe" about conditions, with no idea of where to start to reform things. They know that going to the polls tends to be a meaningless gesture, in which if they know the candidates at all they will usually be choosing between two evils or two mediocrities instead of between a good and an evil or between two goods.

Making Democracy Work. This sense of impotence is the chief disease of the body politic today. Steps must be taken to restore it to health and vitality, if democracy is to have a fair test and show what it can really do. We must make democracy work. But how? There is much earnest discussion on this question. From it all we offer here for consideration a number of suggestions:

(1) We must get away from the notion that politics is dirty and that a decent person will have nothing to do with a political machine. Instead, we ought to seek out the nearest political

organization with which we care to affiliate, get our friends to go with us, and wrest control of the machine from those who seek only to profit from politics and not to serve the community. Also any attempts to restore neighborhood life, to build up community centers, to get together in "town meetings," etc., should be supported. Women especially, since they often have considerable leisure time, ought to devote themselves to this task of revitalizing democracy. And all professional people, including nurses, who have an important stake in honest and efficient government, should abandon their previous aloof attitude and plunge into the midst of politics.

(2) In order to rid politics of job-hunters and job-holders who will do the bidding of political bosses, who wield power by promising and getting jobs for party workers, we must support all movements to establish the merit system, or civil service, in the selection of government employees. The League of Women Voters has made the extension of civil service one of the main planks in its platform for the nation and there are also other civic bodies which are lending their support. Nurses who have worked in county or city hospitals in which the business functions are controlled by politicians as a part of their spoils system, know the importance of establishing civil service.

(3) We must change state constitutions and municipal charters so that they will provide for the election of fewer officials. Democracy does not essentially require the election of a large number of persons. Rather this destroys democracy by putting too great a strain upon the knowledge and ability of the voter. It gives power to the political machine, which takes advantage of the confusion of the voter. If only a few legislative and policy-forming officials were elected and all the rest appointed under civil-service regulations, voting would be much simpler and more intelligent. This movement to substitute the "short ballot" for the present absurdly long ballot should be promoted by all of us who want to make democracy work.

(4) A final suggestion needs more explanation. It concerns the importance of the press in modern democracy. Political equality means not merely equality of opportunity to participate

in party organizations but also equality of opportunity to influence public opinion. Now in earlier days of the Republic, when even New York City was scarcely more than a village, the owner of a newspaper did not have much advantage over any other citizen in controlling public opinion, for anyone who wanted to counteract the influence of a newspaper could do it through personal contacts and speech-making. But today, when newspapers have circulations of hundreds of thousands, what chance has the individual voter against such power? And when we consider, too, how one can inherit a fortune and use it to buy political influence by purchasing a big city newspaper, it is obvious that democracy breaks down here.

There are several ways of restoring political influence to a more equal, or at least more meritorious basis. One is to equalize wealth and incomes as much as possible so that no one can inherit enough money or earn enough money to give him a controlling block of stock in a large newspaper. Secondly, when we become fully conscious of the power vested in the ownership of newspapers, we may see the importance of joining in cooperative enterprises by which we can own our own newspapers. For example, labor unions complain about the unfairness of the capitalistic press, as they style it. Yet think how many newspapers they could buy up if each of their 10,000,000 members would sacrifice $1 a year for this purpose! Thirdly, it would be just as logical for wealthy men to endow newspapers as to endow colleges, since newspapers are probably even more important as educational institutions for the general public, at least in the short run. If some newspapers were controlled by a board of trustees, as colleges and universities are, there would be fewer cities in which the only newspaper is the plaything of some one owner. Finally, newswriters themselves may exert a wholesome control over the press through insistence upon merit as the basis of hiring and advancing members of newspaper staffs and upon professional standards in the selection, emphasis, and reporting of news. Great advance has already been made in the past two decades through the quiet pressure of professionalism upon the owners of newspapers, and still further democratization may be expected in the future.

Liberty

A society could conceivably be democratic in so far as providing equality of educational and vocational opportunity and yet be ruled by an administrative hierarchy, with power vested only in the hands of those who have worked up to the higher positions. Such was the social organization which Plato described in his utopia, the *Republic.* It was a perfectly just system (for each did the work which he could best do, and the rulers, being all-wise, ruled) but not completely democratic, first, because it was not based upon the ultimate power of the people, and, secondly, because freedom of speech and writing was in part not allowed. Since no rulers are all-wise, democracy requires more than justice—it requires popular sovereignty and freedom of speech and press and assemblage. Indeed, the former cannot really function without the latter, for citizens cannot vote intelligently unless they have full access to the facts and full opportunity to influence and be influenced by others.

Theory of Knowledge Underlying Doctrine of Liberty. This phase of democracy is based upon a theory of knowledge which assumes that the truth is more likely to be attained in the long run in a society of persons who have the privilege of saying or writing whatever they please. It assumes that in a free competition of ideas the truth will win out. Since truth is consistency with the broadest possible human experience, the best way to attain truth is to make our experience as broad as possible, which means hearing and discussing opinions which we think are false as well as those which we think are true.

Freedom of speech and press is also based upon a historical generalization. We have observed that progress has been delayed, sometimes probably for centuries, by suppression of views which were thought to be harmful, while in the modern age in countries where freedom has existed the greatest scientific, political, and moral progress has been made. Even if a particular idea or book or play seems very dangerous, it cannot be half so dangerous as censorship would be.

Liberty and Progress. Political freedom is the keystone to all other freedoms and is indispensable for the trial-and-error process which intelligent beings employ. We can lose all other freedoms without great danger as long as we have political freedom which permits us to argue in favor of restoring these other freedoms. But, once we give up freedom of speech and press, there is no way of correcting that mistake except by illegal and perhaps violent means. Freedom to advocate change in government, religion, morals or any other phase of culture is *strategic* for progress. John Milton gave eloquent expression to this democratic doctrine three centuries ago when he said, "Give me the liberty to know, to utter, and to argue freely according to conscience, above all other liberties." And Voltaire wrote, "I do not agree with a word that you say, but I will defend to the death your right to say it."

Exceptions to Freedom of Press. Ought a democracy ever to make an exception to the rule of political freedom? Obviously in war we do make an exception and introduce censorship of the press. It is notable, however, that especially during the second world war both England and the United States had a remarkable record of maintaining political freedom in everything which did not directly involve military strategy. Only news which might be of military value to the enemy was suppressed. Editors and citizens were free to criticize the government. And Congress could have repealed military censorship regulations at any time if it had desired to do so. This freedom was absolutely essential to maintaining civilian morale, for we had reached a point in our cultural development in which we would not cooperate fully unless we were "in" on things and were treated like responsible, mature beings.

Many persons believe that democracies ought not to tolerate revolutionaries who advocate the violent overthrow of the government. It is agreed by all that if these revolutionaries came into power they would immediately silence us democratic liberals. So, it is argued, why should we allow them to use our democratic Bill of Rights for the very purpose of destroying it? This misses the main point of liberalism. Freedom of speech is granted to revolutionaries because any abridgment of the freedom of speech opens the door to complete suppression of speech; hence true democrats do not want to get into the habit of suppressing opinions with which they do not agree. Also open-minded democrats want to profit by whatever criticisms revolutionaries may have to make of our society.

Our courts in their most enlightened decisions have made a distinction between (a) advocating revolution in a general way and (b) inciting persons to immediate acts of violence—the former being legal, the latter being illegal. Some deplore this. Others consider it the wisest policy to pursue when a democracy is as well established as ours. A democracy which had a bare majority might be justified in placing severe restrictions upon the enemies of the democratic regime, but in a country like ours it is absurd for an overwhelming majority to be afraid to let a handful of revolutionaries express themselves, especially since suppressing them only gives them precisely the publicity and sympathy which they seek.

Vocational Freedom. In addition to political liberty, a democratic culture provides as much vocational freedom for individuals as is practicable. Our rule is to give the individual as wide a range of choice as possible in selecting and pursuing a career. In every business and professional organization our ideal should be to give everyone from the lowest position to the highest the broadest range of discretion consistent with efficiency, so that every citizen will have the self-respecting feeling which comes from making decisions.

Personal Liberty. In personal affairs the democratic doctrine of liberty means leaving as many things as possible in the realm of individual taste rather than making them matters of morals. John Stuart Mill, an English philosopher of the nineteenth century, in his *Essay on Liberty*, gave classical expression to the principle of personal liberty, when he said that we ought to exert neither legal nor moral pressure upon anyone unless we are sure that he is doing something essentially harmful to ourselves or others. In other words, we should be broadly tolerant of the conduct of others unless we can show clearly how *someone else's* happiness is being injured by it. This does not mean that we should be indifferent morally to unwise conduct of life on the part of the individual but that we should be very cautious about condemning others when their conduct apparently injures only themselves. There is always the possibility that we may be mistaken about its injurious effects on the person himself or that our judgment may be based upon prejudice or superstition.

Religious Freedom. Religious freedom is not an independent element in democratic liberalism but is derived from the basic liberties we have already discussed. In so far as religion involves the expression of ideas, then it is important for cultural progress that everyone be free to say and write whatever he believes. And in so far as religion consists in worship and ceremonial observances, then it is a matter of personal taste which does not harm others and therefore ought to be tolerated. Freedom of religion, however, does not mean the right to act in ways that are directly injurious to others. For example, human sacrifice would not be tolerated on the ground that it is a religious rite. And courts have sometimes protected children against parents who have refused on religious grounds to give them medical attention. That, at any rate, indicates the theoretical limits of the right to religious freedom. Actually, in this country we have been so eager to prevent the spread of religious intolerance that we have permitted a good deal of loss of life and health in the name of religion. This policy has met with objection. Yet public opinion in general has considered the courts and legislatures wise in not exercising the full rights of the state to protect its members against harm. It is better that the law remain a "blunt instrument," as one jurist has called it, rather than that the floodgates of religious intolerance should be opened.

International Democracy

Our discussion of democratic ideals has chiefly centered about our own nation. Events leading up to the war, however, have shown us that we cannot enjoy democracy at home without sharing at least some of it with other nations. This does not mean that we should impose our form of government upon them but that we should give them access to the resources and the trade which is necessary for a high level of living. Also we have learned that we must abandon our isolationism and nationalism at least enough to join other non-aggressive nations in policing the world so that never again will peace and freedom be threatened. With prosperity and peace assured to other lands, their governments will have a chance to evolve in a democratic direction, as ours has. It is only insecurity and crisis that cause people to lose themselves in nationalistic frenzy and place their lives and fortunes in the hands of a dictator. And, incidentally, we ourselves shall have a much better opportunity to improve our own democracy if we do not have to suffer the disorganization of war every generation.

Humanitarian Outlook of Nurses. Nurses need no urging to think in terms of humanity rather than in terms of the narrow limits of one nation. Nursing, like science and art, has been international in outlook almost since its beginning in modern times. We can, therefore, look to nurses, as well as to all other persons of intelligence and good will, to work for the new era of peace and freedom and brotherhood of which J. A. Symonds sings prophetically in his hymn, *The Human Outlook:*

> These things shall be! a loftier race
>   Than e'er the world hath known, shall rise
> With flame of freedom in their souls,
>   And light of science in their eyes.
>
> They shall be gentle, brave, and strong,
>   To spill no drop of blood, but dare
> All that may plant man's lordship firm
>   On earth, and fire, and sea, and air.
>
> Nation with nation, land with land,
>   Unarmed shall live as comrades free;
> In every heart and brain shall throb
>   The pulse of one fraternity.
>
> These things—they are no dreams—shall be
>   For happier men when we are gone;
> Those golden days for them shall dawn,
>   Transcending aught we gaze upon.

Study Questions

1. What sort of living did the average family in this country have before the second world war?
2. Why were we able to employ almost everyone during the war but not previously?
3. What good rules of individual economy do not apply to the nation as a whole?

4. Ought we to try to pay back the national debt? Under what conditions should we try to stabilize (not increase further) the national debt?

5. How does taxation help modern capitalism to function?

6. Ought prices to rise when the public has greater purchasing power? Why or why not?

7. Why did international trade break down during the thirties? What was the underlying pressure for war?

8. What increase in the nation's health budget would be required in order to give adequate medical care to everyone?

9. Describe the following plans for financing more adequate medical and hospital services: (a) group hospitalization insurance; (b) prepayment of medical services; (c) compulsory health insurance; (d) state medicine.

10. What are the advantages and dangers of state medicine?

11. Would nurses be better off under a system of state medicine?

12. What is the explanation of the fact that we are often represented by mediocre men in legislatures and in congress?

13. Mention four things that need to be done to improve political democracy?

14. What is the difference between a just state and a democratic state?

15. Ought exceptions ever to be made to the rule of freedom of speech and of the press?

16. What was John Stuart Mill's formula for personal liberty? What argument could there be in applying the formula?

17. What should we do to encourage the spread of democracy throughout the world?

Questions for Thought and Discussion

1. Do you agree with this statement: "We believe in freedom but this means the freedom to do what is right"?

2. What type of international organization do you think will be productive of the greatest peace and prosperity throughout the world?

3. List a few scientific discoveries or inventions which have reached only a limited portion of the population of the United States.
4. What are the principal causes of the lag in applying scientific knowledge for the improvement of life?
5. What sort of gifts or loans to other countries might result ultimately in the raising of our standard of living? What sort of gifts or loans would not have that effect?
6. How does it happen that there are efficient public health departments in some cities and states that have otherwise inefficient and corrupt governments?
7. Do you believe that a system of nursing insurance to cover the cost of private nursing should be added to medical and hospital insurance? Why?
8. What measures would you advocate for providing adequate medical care for the American people?
9. Very many rural sections in the United States have grossly inadequate nursing care as compared with urban sections. In your opinion, should the nursing profession assume any responsibility for more equal distribution of nursing service?

Books to Read

Bellamy, Edward: *Looking Backward.* Cleveland. World Publishing Co. Tower Books. 1945.

Chase, Stuart: *Where's the Money Coming From?* New York. The Twentieth Century Fund. 1943.

Federal Council of Churches of Christ: *Social Justice and Economic Reconstruction.*

Hansen, Alvin H.: *After the War—Full Employment, Post-war Planning.* U. S. Government Printing Office. 1942.

Hoover, Herbert, and Gibson, Hugh: *The Problem of Lasting Peace.* New York. Doubleday, Doran. 1942.

Laski, Harold J.: *Where Do We Go from Here?* New York. Viking Press. 1940.

Mill, John Stuart: *Utilitarianism, Liberty and Representative Government.* Everyman's Library. 1926.

Mumford, Lewis: *Culture of Cities*. New York. Harcourt, Brace. 1938.

Survey Graphic: issue entitled "Fitness for Freedom." March, 1942.

Tufts, J. H.: *America's Social Morality*. New York. Henry Holt. 1933; Chapters IX to XII.

Willkie, Wendell L.: *One World*. New York. Simon and Schuster. 1943.

Index

Nursing, art of, 41
care, distribution of, 233
civilization and, 1, 6
education, 13
future of, 1 ff.
government agencies and, 12
incomes and sex inequality, 7
industrial, 13
institutional, 10
intelligence in, 46 ff.
a practical training for life, 15
preparation for, 23
private, 9 f.
income in, 10
profession, incomes in, 7 ff.
growth of, 6 f.
worldwide humanitarianism
and, 113
public health, 11
service and underprivileged, 5
special fields of, 14
temperament for, 22

OATH of Hippocrates, 164
Obedience to orders and rules, 41
undiscriminating, 77
Objectivity as part of professional
attitude, 39
Office of Indian Affairs, 12
Old age pensions, 178
One-price system for nurses, 168
Opportunities in nursing, 8 ff.
Orders, doctor's, obedience to,
160 ff.
Organizations, professional, 63 ff.,
71 ff.
student, 63 ff.

PAIN, submission to, 121
Parental feeling, expression of, as
basic need, 126

Parenthood, planned, 91, 184
Parliamentary law, 65 ff.
keynote to democracy, toler-
ance, rationality, and prog-
ress, 66
Pasteur, early opposition to
methods of, 86
Patient, care of, nurse's responsi-
bility in, 38
dying wishes of, moral respon-
sibility regarding, 61
intimacy with, 164 f.
Patient's effects, loss of, subject
to legal action, 58
Peace problems, nurse and, 98
Pensions, mother's, 178
old age, 178
Perpetua, 180
Perseus, shield of, 19
Personality, 22
Pessimism, 175 f.
Physical ability, 23
Physicians, unscrupulous, 158–159
Plato, 135, 152, 221, 243
Political system, wrong, 240
Politics, discussion of, with
patient, 165
participation in, by professional
people, 241 f.
Practical considerations in evalu-
ating conduct, 221
Pregnancy, ectopic, interruption
of, 187
interruption of, incidental to
life-saving measure, 187
Preparation for nursing, 23 ff.
Press, freedom of, 243 ff.
and democracy, 241 f.
Private nursing, 9 f.
Professional appearance, 40
attitude and a democratic
manner, 217 f.
with patients, 42

Titles in This Series

14   Annette Fiske. *First Fifty Years of the Waltham Training School for Nurses*. New York, 1984. BOUND WITH Alfred Worcester. "The Shortage of Nurses—Reminiscences of Alfred Worcester '83." *Harvard Medical Alumni Bulletin 23*, 1949.

15   Virginia Henderson et al. *Nursing Studies Index, 1900–1959*. Philadelphia, 1963, 1966, 1970, 1972.

16   Darlene Clark Hine, editor. *Black Women in Nursing: An Anthology of Historical Sources*.

17   Ellen N. LaMotte. *The Tuberculosis Nurse*. New York, 1915.

18   Barbara Melosh, editor. *American Nurses in Fiction: An Anthology of Short Stories*.

19   Mary Adelaide Nutting. *A Sound Economic Basis for Schools of Nursing*. New York, 1926.

20   Sara E. Parsons. *Nursing Problems and Obligations*. Boston, 1916.

21   Juanita Redmond. *I Served on Bataan*. Philadelphia, 1943.

22   Susan Reverby, editor. *The East Harlem Health Center Demonstration: An Anthology of Pamphlets*.

23   Isabel Hampton Robb. *Educational Standards for Nurses*. Cleveland, 1907.

24   Sister M. Theophane Shoemaker. *History of Nurse-Midwifery in the United States*. Washington, D.C., 1947.

25   Isabel M. Stewart. *Education of Nurses*. New York, 1943.

26   Virginia S. Thatcher. *History of Anesthesia with Emphasis on the Nurse Specialist*. Philadelphia, 1953.

27   Adah H. Thoms. *Pathfinders—A History of the Progress of Colored Graduate Nurses*. New York, 1929.

28   Clara S. Weeks-Shaw. *A Text-Book of Nursing for the Use of Training Schools, Families, and Private Students*. New York, 1885.

29   Writers Program of the WPA in Kansas, compilers. *Lamps on the Prairie: A History of Nursing in Kansas*. Topeka, 1942.